PRACTICE OF TRADITIONAL AND COMPLEMENTARY MEDICINE AMONG HEALTH PROFESSIONALS IN MALAYSIA

Associate Professor Dr. Magfiret Abdulveli Bozlar; PhD
Professor Dr. Syed Mohamed Aljunid; PhD

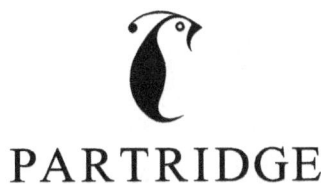

PARTRIDGE

Copyright © 2020 by DR. MAGFIRET A. BOZLAR,
PROF. DR. SYED ALJUNID.

ISBN:	Softcover	978-1-5437-5721-7
	eBook	978-1-5437-5722-4

All rights reserved. No part of this book may be used or reproduced by any means, graphic, electronic, or mechanical, including photocopying, recording, taping or by any information storage retrieval system without the written permission of the author except in the case of brief quotations embodied in critical articles and reviews.

Because of the dynamic nature of the Internet, any web addresses or links contained in this book may have changed since publication and may no longer be valid. The views expressed in this work are solely those of the author and do not necessarily reflect the views of the publisher, and the publisher hereby disclaims any responsibility for them.

Print information available on the last page.

To order additional copies of this book, contact
Toll Free 800 101 2657 (Singapore)
Toll Free 1 800 81 7340 (Malaysia)
orders.singapore@partridgepublishing.com

www.partridgepublishing.com/singapore

CONTENTS

Acknowledgement ix

Chapter 1 Introduction 1

    Background 1
    Definition 6
    Classification of Traditional and
        Complementary Medicine in Malaysia 7
    Current Status of Traditional and
        Complementary Medicine in Malaysia 22
    Traditional and Complementary Medicine
        Integrated Hospitals 29
    Traditional and Complementary Medicine
        Overview and its Importance in Malaysia 30
    Potential Benefits of this Study 31
    General Issues 32
    Research Questions 33
    Research Justification 34
    Objectives 36
    Reaseach Hypotheses 37

Chapter 2 Literature Review 38

    The Practice of Traditional and
        Complementary Medicine 38
    Conceptual Framework 47

Chapter 3 Methodology 49
- Introduction 49
- Background of the Study Location 49
- Study Design 51
- Study Locations and Population 51
- Sampling Frame 51
- Sampling Unit 51
- Sampling Method 52
- Sample Size 52
- Inclusion And Exclusion Criteria 53
- Study Instruments 53
- Sampling for Qualitative Study 57
- Study Variables 61
- Operational Definition of Variables 61
- Data Collection and Analysis 65

Chapter 4 Results 67
- Socio-Demographic Factors, Knowledge, Attitude, Practice of T&CM, and Reasons for Practicing or Not Practicing T&CM 67
- Relationship Between Socio-Demographic Characteristics Of Health Professionals and Their Use of T&CM and T&CM Referral to Patients and Family 87
- Multivariable Logistic Regression Analysis to Predict the Use and Referral to T&CM among Health Professionals 140
- Qualitative Study on Practice of T&CM 160
- Summary 171

Chapter 5 Discussion 173

The Rate of T&CM Use and Referral...................... 174
Modalities of T&CM 174
Association Between Use/Referral of T&CM
   and Socio-Demographic Characteristics of
   Health Professionals 176
Association Between the Use of T&CM
   Among Health Professionals and
   Knowledge Regarding T&CM........................... 192
Association Between Use of T&CM among
   Health Professionals and Attitude Towards
   T&CM 194
Association Between Use of T&CM among
   Health Professionals and Perception
   About Education/Training in T&CM 199
Reason for Precticing and Not Practicing T&CM 201
Factors Influencing The T&CM Use/
   Recommendation.. 202
Strength of the Study.. 203
Study Limitation 203

Chapter 6 Conclusion and Recommendations 204

Conclusion 204
Recommendations.. 209

References 211

ACKNOWLEDGEMENT

In the name of Allah, the most gracious and the most merciful. First of all, Alhamdulillah and praise to Allah for grace and his mercy in giving me the health and strength to complete this book. First of all, we express our sincere and heartfelt acknowledgements the following individuals: Imranjan, son of Dr. Magfiret Abdulveli Bozlar and her husband Ahmet Bozlar, her brothers Muhammad Yusup Akhun, Yasin Akhun, Memtimin akhun and sister Ayjamal and Sahipjamal who understands and encourages her. Without their support she would not have completed this book. She would like to express her deep gratitude to her late father for his love and constant encouragement and motivation. He taught her the value of education, a value needed to pursue her academic goals. The word "gratitude" is not enough to convey her profound appreciation and respect to her late mother for giving her the gift of happiness and for working so hard to get her a good education. Her love, encouragement and support gave her the spirit to continue learning in the area of Traditional Medicine, the profession of her grandfather, great grandfather and so on.

We are so grateful to Associate Professor Dr. Zaleha Md Isa from National University of Malaysia for suggesting the research, her continuous interest, her generous guidance, her constructive criticism, never-ceasing opportunities for insightful discussion and her invaluable supervision throughout the course of the study. We would like to convey our deep appreciation and heartfelt gratitude to Dr. Sima Barmania, Assistant Professor Dr. Nametjan Memet, and also Tan Sri Dr. Mohamed Salleh Mohamed Yasin, Professor Nur Hassim Ismail and all the Medical Research Secretariat Officers (UKMMC) staff for their support, kindness and friendly advice. Special thanks are also extended to the Members of The Medical Research and Ethics Committee of UKM and also the Secretariat Office. We also wish to extend our gratitude to Traditional and Complementary Medicine Division, Ministry of Health, Malaysia. Words cannot adequately express the feeling of appreciation and gratitude we have for those who helped us to complete this field of study in Malaysia. We are deeply grateful to the all the Departments of the University Kebangsaan Malaysia Medical Center, Hospital Putrajaya, Hospital Sultanah Nur Zahirah, Hospital Duchess of Kent and Sarawak General Hospital for their active participation, continual discussion, and valuable assistance in the collecting of data. Lastly, We wish to express our sincere gratitude to all participants of this study in the mentioned five hospitals in Malaysia. Without their assistance and generous cooperation this work could not have been fulfilled.

LIST OF ABBREVIATIONS

AIDS	Acquired immune deficiency syndrome
BBT	Biological-Based Medicine
CAM	Complementary and Alternative Medicine
CAMs	Complementary and Alternative Medicines
CMDs	Complementary Medicine doctors
CM	Conventional Medicine
CZ	Czech
CME	Continuing Medical Education
CHBQ	Complementary Medicine Health Belief Questioner
DCA	Drug Control Authority
DGH	City district general hospital
PhD	Doctor of Philosophy
SARS	Severe acute respiratory syndrome
RM	Malaysian Ringgit
R&D	Research and development
HIV	Human immunodeficiency virus
HMRC	Herbal Medicine Research Center
$US	US Dollar
NHP	Natural Health Products
NCCAM	National Center for Complementary and Alternative Medicine
NHPH	Natural Health Products Directorate
NGO's	Non Governmental Organizations
NCTs	Non-conventional therapies
NHW	Non-Hispanic women
MD	Medical doctors
MQA	Ministry of Education and Malaysian Qualifications Agency

MOH	Ministry of Health
IMR	Institute for Health System Research
IHSR	Institute for Health System Research
IRPA	Intensified Research in Priority Areas
OMDs	Oriental medical doctors
T&CM	Traditional and Complementary Medicine
TM	Traditional Medicine
TCM	Traditional Chinese Medicine
TM/CAM	Traditional Medicine/ Complementary and Alternative Medicine
T&CMD	Traditional and Complementary Medicine Division
UNESCO	United Nations Educational, Scientific and Cultural Organization
USA	United States of America
UKMMC	Universiti Kebangsaan Malaysia Medical Center
U.S	United States
UK	United Kingdom
UMMC	University Maryland Medical Center
WHO	World Health Organization
WM	Western Medicine
WMDs	Western Medicine doctors
WMD-CMDs	Western Medicine doctors and Complementary Medicine doctors
WM-T&CM	Western Medicine and Traditional & Complementary Medicine
KAP	Knowledge, Attitude and Practice
NHPD	Natural Health Products Directorate

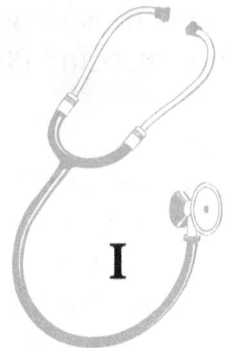

I

INTRODUCTION

BACKGROUND

Malaysia is situated in Southeast Asia, neighbored by Thailand in the north, Indonesia in the south, and the Philippines in the east. It consists of thirteen states and three federal territories and has a total landmass of 330,803 square kilometres (127,720 sq mi) separated by the South China Sea into two similarly sized regions, Peninsular Malaysia and East Malaysia (Malaysian Borneo) (Wikipedia). Malaysia is the 66th largest country by total land area. It is a multi-racial country which comprises of different ethnic groups such as, Malays, Chinese, Indian and indigenous people with a population over 30 million (Wikipedia). Kuala Lumpur, the capital of Malaysia is located in the Federal Territory, which is one of three Malaysian Federal Territories, surrounded by the state of Selangor, on the central west coast of Malaysia Peninsular. Fifteen decade ago, Malaysia was almost completely covered with jungle. Today, it is one of the richest and best developed country in Asia. Malaysia's economy was ranked 6th in Asia and 20th in the world in 2014-2015 (Source: IMF & World Bank 2012 – 2014).

Traditional and Complementary Medicine (T&CM) has been gaining acknowledgement and acceptance all over the world including Malaysia. It is the most invaluable treasure of the oriental civilization and has been developed over the course of thousands of years in the quest for human wellbeing (Chaudhury & Rafei 2001; Eisenberg et al. 1998). Almost all Asian nations have developed a certain system of traditional medicine based on theories, beliefs and experiences indigenous to different cultures that are used to maintain health, as well as to prevent, diagnose, improve or treat physical and mental illness (WHO 2013; Koumpouros & Birbas 2013). Malaysia is a multi-ethnic, multicultural country that has rich various traditional practice modalities.

The primary health care recognizes the importance of T&CM. It is a known fact that majorities of people in developing countries still depend on the use of traditional medicine for their health care needs (Odugbemi 2008; Tindle et al. 2005). T&CM is already widely used by most countries especially herbal medicine; therefore expenditure of T&CM is getting higher year by year. However, not more than half of the populations of developed countries and as high as 80% people used in developing countries use traditional medicine (WHO 2000; Shmueli 2004). Between 70–95% of the population rely on traditional medicines for primary care in majority of the developing countries especially in Asia, Africa, Latin America and Middle East (Molly & Xiaorui 2011).

PRACTICE OF TRADITIONAL AND COMPLEMENTARY MEDICINE AMONG HEALTH PROFESSIONALS IN MALAYSIA

In Germany, 80% of physicians prescribed phytomedicines, which account for 27% of all over the counter medicines and more than half of adults first turn to natural remedies for treatment of illness. The same trend applies to other European countries with Canada 70%, France 49%, Australia 48% and Belgium 38% as regular uses of complementary and alternative medicine (CAM) (Payyappallimana 2009).

WHO estimates that half of Canadians and more than two third of French have tried CAM which often includes herbal remedies (Aschwanden 2001). In the USA, it was estimated in 1990 that at least one in three Americans utilized one CAM, and in a 1997 follow-up study, the percentage of CAM patients had increased from 33.8% to 42% of the U.S population (Eisenberg et al. 1998; Molly & Xiaorui 2011). Every year plant based anti-cancer drugs save at least 30,000 lives only in U.S. The large majority of people in Africa use traditional medicine regularly. In Sub-Saharan Africa for example, 85% of the population go to traditional healers (Hanssen et al 2005).

In Brazil, nearly 90% of cancer patients used TM/CAM. In Ghana, Mali, Nigeria and Zambia, herbal medicines are administered at home as first-aid treatment for 60% of children with high fever caused by malaria (UNESCO 2010). India is one of the richest countries in the world in the field of ethnobotanical knowledge. Around more than two thirds of the population in India relies on these systems for primary health care. The proportion of use of plants in the different Indian systems of medicine is: Ayurveda 2000, Siddha 1300,

Unani 1000, Homeopathy 800, Tibetan 500, Modern 200 and folk 4500 (Barnes et al. 2008; Pandey et al. 2008).

T&CM including herbal medicine has grown substantially in public awareness and became one of the prime agenda of medical researchers across the world. In China, traditional herbal medicine played a prominent role in the strategy to contain and treat severe acute respiratory syndromes (SARS) (WHO 2008). A traditional herbal medicine, Africa Flower, has been used for decades to treat wasting symptoms associated with HIV (WHO 2008; Abuduli 2011; Buono et al. 2001; Tilburt & Kaptchukb 2008). Uyghur herbal medicine succeeded in treatment of hepatitis B in Xinjiang nearly 30 years ago (Abuduli 2011).

Many hope that traditional herbal medicine research will play a critical role in global health (Tilburt & Kaptchuk 2008). Interest in practices of T&CM has grown considerably in recent years. In the modern era, some sophisticatedly developed medical systems still in wide application in treating certain chronicle ailments. T&CM is not only viewed as having clinically beneficial but is also generally believed to be safe (Mills 2006; Shih et al. 2010).

T&CM developed before its inception and it is not easily understood by modern medicine, often due to the lack of scientific evaluation (WHO 2000). Practices and forms of traditional medicine, however, vary greatly from country to country. The role of traditional medicine is also different among countries and areas of the region. Although T&CM may not be fully explicable by modern science at the moment,

PRACTICE OF TRADITIONAL AND
COMPLEMENTARY MEDICINE AMONG HEALTH
PROFESSIONALS IN MALAYSIA

its further development and a possible merger with modern medicine in the future should not be ruled out (WHO 2000).

Being aware of the important role played by T&CM in preventive, promotive and curative aspect of health care for large populations, especially in developing countries; WHO has been increasingly supportive in tapping its full potential and wide application in various countries. T&CM including herbal medicine is going to be a new and fast growing industry at an international level and continues to be patronized by the community on treating the disease and preserving well-being (National Policy of Traditional and Complementary Medicine, 2001).

Different types of T&CM treatments are applied and practiced by the public increases but ignorance about T&CM poses a communication gap between public health and the healthcare profession. Most western-trained physicians are ignorant of the benefits and risks of this healthcare modality and assessment of acceptance and knowledge would identify appropriate intervention strategies to improve physician-patient communication in this area (Clement et al. 2005).

About two thirds of Malaysia is covered in forest and some forests are believed to be 130 million years old (Wikipedia). More than 35,000 plants have been reported to have been used for medical purposes in various human cultures around the world (Taid et al. 2014). There are around 12,000 plants and there are many medicinal plants that have been used for thousands of years (Wikipedia). It is recorded that not less than 1,300 plants have been used in traditional medicine in Malaysia (Jantan 2004).

Today, because of the therapeutic efficacy of many of those herbs, they can be found in herbal products and as part of the traditional Malaysian health care system. Many herbs have been use by Malays, Chinese, Indians, aboriginal people (Orang Asli) and other ethnic groups in such as Kadazan, Dusun, Iban and Bajau in Sabah and Sarawak areas.

DEFINITION

T&CM is a controversial area with even definition and term of the T&CM differing between one country to another and between one region to another. Therefore, while adopting the WHO definition of traditional medicine, emphasis is laid on the geographical diversity and variety of its practices (UNESCO 2010). That is why, T&CM is called by different names such as traditional medicine, complementary and alternative medicine (CAM), complementary medicine, alternative medicine, or sometimes it is called by its specific name such as Ayurveda, Unani, Homeopathy and Siddha in India; Chinese, Uyghur, Tibetan and Mongolian medicine in China. In Malaysia, it has been called Traditional and Complementary Medicine (T&CM). T&CM is also called by its specific name. T&CM is a term generally used to describe the practice of medicine which is not of the conventional scientific medicine (Abuduli et al. 2011; Zhang et al. 2011).

WHO defines Traditional Medicine as diverse health practices, approaches, and knowledge and believes that cooperating plants, animal and/or mineral-based medicines, spiritual therapies, manual techniques and exercises applied singularly or in combination to maintain well-being, as well as to treat, diagnose or prevent illness (WHO 2005). The terms complementary/alternative/non-conventional medicine are used interchangeably with traditional medicine in some countries (WHO 2005; Kim et al. 2002).

CAM refers to a broad set of healthcare practices that are not part of a country's own tradition and not integrated into the dominant healthcare system. Other terms were sometimes used to describe these healthcare practices, including 'natural medicine', 'non-conventional medicine' and 'holistic medicine' (Chen & Hu 2006; WHO 2000).

According to the definition by the Ministry of Health (MOH), Malaysia, T&CM means a form of health-related practice designed to prevent, treat, and/or manage illness and/ or preserve the mental and physical well-being of individuals and it includes practices such as traditional Malay medicine, traditional Chinese medicine, traditional Indian medicine, homeopathy, complementary therapies and Islamic medicine however, it excludes medical or dental practices by registered medical or dental practitioners (MOH 2004).

CLASSIFICATION OF TRADITIONAL AND COMPLEMENTARY MEDICINE IN MALAYSIA

Traditional and Complementary Medicine is classified into six groups in Malaysia. These are Islamic medical practice, traditional Malay medicine, traditional Chinese medicine, traditional Indian medicine, Homeopathy and Complementary Medicine. T&CM is adapted the concept of therapeutic and wellness.

1. Islamic Medical Practice

The Ministry of Health has agreed to add Islamic medicine in the Traditional and Complementary Medicine (T&CM) Bill 2012 after it was agreed by the Jabatan Kemajuan Islam Malaysia (Malaysia Islamic Development Department) and all the Islamic religious departments. However, Islamic Medical practice is relatively small in Malaysia. It is practiced by private hospitals which are mainly located in Kuala Lumpur, Terengganu and Kelantan. Most of the Muslims believe and practice Islamic medicine in Malaysia (Traditional and Complementary Medicine Division 2011).

Islamic Medical Practice (Ruqyah) refers to prayer therapy by practitioners during treatments. The effort of seeking treatment for physical and spiritual ailments; done by a Muslim who is knowledgeable and skilled in treatment methods using Quranic verses, Hadith, the practices of the pious and righteous scholars, and of the venerated religious teacher (Sabry & Vohra 2013; Traditional and Complementary Medicine Division 2011).

Many Muslims prefer to consume honey, grapes, black seed or black seed oil, olive oil, dates, and zamzam water or special water where the Qur'an has been recited on and blowed into water; this kind of healing water is available in some hospitals' shop.

Most of the patients rely on Islamic healing, especially Muslim cancer patients seek Islamic healing practice and demand for Islamic healing therapies has increased especially among cancer patients in Malaysia (Yatim et al; Suhami et al. 2014).

The recitation of Quran verses as a main method with du'a & sunnah salat and combination of herbs with recitation of Quran verses, du'a and healing water are popular among Muslim women with cancer (Suhami et al. 2014). Black magic, misusing of the Holy Quran (physically and Quranic verses), bedah batin (virtual surgery) and use of azimat (amulet), tangkal (talisman), susuk (charm needles) are prohibited in Islamic medicine (Traditional and Complementary Medicine Division 2011).

2. **Traditional Malay Medicine**

Traditional Malay medicine is a field of knowledge and practices which are indigenous to Malay culture that cover aspects of health and healing which are practiced from generation to generation (Globinmed 2015). It is inherited through oral traditions, written forms and practices, and believes of the Malay race. Principles of Malay traditional medicine is based on the Greek model of four elements and four humours which are similar to Uyghur and Unani medicine. Traditional healers use various methods of treatments for patients. The treatment of ailments uses a holistic approach, involving physical, spiritual, mental, emotional and behavioral factors (Ikram & Ghani 2015). Malay medicine is influenced by other practices of Indonesian, Chinese, Indian and indigenous people (Orang asli) traditional medicines.

Traditional Malay medicine includes Malay traditional herbal medicine, Malay massage (urut Melayu), Malay postnatal care, cupping (bekam), indigenous massage, male vitality treatment, female health treatment, Malay traditional treatment for sinus (rawatan resdung) etc. A survey shows that 52 plant species are used in traditional medicine by the Malay villagers and the most common plant parts used in the preparation of Malay herbal medicine are leaves, roots and fruits. Malay herbs can be collected from home garden or forests (Ong et al. 2011).

Malay massage (Urut Melayu) is used for post stroke patients in T&CM integrated hospitals in Malaysia. There are many post stroke patients who receive the therapeutic massage and acupuncture therapy from T&CM units of the T&CM integrated hospitals. I interviewed some post stroke patients regarding the T&CM treatments and services in 2012. They were satisfied from the treatments but did not agree to get recommendations from western trained doctors who do not have knowledge about T&CM for the T&CM treatment and also they all want to increase the duration of massage therapy. Almost all of them said they got the therapeutic massage from private massage centers because of the difficulties of getting the recommendations from medical doctors most of the time and some of them said they use some herbal remedies as well but they never informed their doctors. Meanwhile, all of them expected to fully integrate T&CM into the Malaysian healthcare system.

A case study shows that a woman who had postpartum stroke received whole body massage for 14 sections in a T&CM

integrated hospital and she improved her speech, fine motor skills and regained her activities for daily living.

Malaysia is blessed with herbal and natural products. Sanggul Fatimah (Anastatica hierochuntica L. or The True Rose Of Jericho) is a very well-known traditional herb. For thousands of years across the Middle East, Asia and Africa, Sanggul Fatimah has been used when pregnant women are in labour (Ghazali 2009). Malay women in Kelantan believed that Sanggul Fatimah tea helps to ease childbirth.

Study shows that one third of pregnant women use herbal medicine. The most commonly used herbs are Sanggul Fatimah 60.1% and coconut oil 35.4% (Sooi & Keng 2013). More than two thirds of women used herbal medicine during labor because of a belief that it may shorten and ease labor. Sanggul Fatimah is used in labor and post labor as it is believed it will enhance good tissue and organ repair (Ghazali 2009).

Kacip Fatimah (Labisia pumila) is one of the famous plants in South East Asian community especially in Malaysia. It is called "queen of plants". Kacip Fatimah is used as a food and beverage. In the Malay community it is considered beneficial to women. It is believed that kacip fatimah is good for easing of childbirth, as a post-partum medication to contract the birth channel, regulation of the menstrual cycle, and alleviation of menstrual symptoms (Ibrahim et al. 2011; Wikipedia 2008).

Ahmad Nazrun Shuid et al. (2011) showed that kacip fatimah has the potential to be utilised as an alternative treatment for postmenopausal osteoporosis. Higher doses of kacip fatimah may be needed to match estrogen in terms of preventing the bone calcium loss (Shuid et al. 2011). A study showed that kacip fatimah extract has tremendous potential as an anti-photoaging cosmetic ingredient (Choi et al. 2011). Another study showed that kacip fatimah increases uterine weight, indicating estrogenic effects, and improves insulin sensitivity and lipid profile in PCOS rats without affecting body composition (Manneras et al. 2009).

Bitter melon (Momordica charantia, bitter gourd, bitter squash) also known as bitter gourd or karela is a unique vegetable or fruit and is used as a food or medicine. It has long been used as herbal remedy for various diseases and ailments including type 2 diabetes (Dans 2007). The fruit contains at least three active substances with anti-diabetic properties, which has been confirmed to have a blood glucose-lowering effect. A. Fuangchan et al. (2011) showed that a 2,000 mg daily dose of bitter melon significantly reduced blood glucose levels among patients with type 2 diabetes. Some other studies have also supported the health benefits of bitter melon for type 2 diabetes (Leung et al. 2009).

Tongkat Ali root or Pasak Bumi (Eurycoma longifolia) is commonly called "Malaysian ginseng". The plant is famous in Malaysia, Indonesia, Thailand, Vietnam and Laos. It is a natural testosterone boosting herb. It has long been used as an aphrodisiac and a remedy for age-related sexual disorders and symptoms of andropause. Tongkat Ali has anti-aging properties and also improves libido, energy, sports performance, reduces stress and weight loss. There are various types of Tongkat Ali products in Malaysia (Talbot et al. 2013).

PRACTICE OF TRADITIONAL AND COMPLEMENTARY MEDICINE AMONG HEALTH PROFESSIONALS IN MALAYSIA

Prickly pear cactus (Opuntia spp or nopal) is also one of the favorite herbs in Malaysia which has been used for type 2 diabetes, high cholesterol, nausea, obesity, alcohol hangover, colitis, diarrhea, and has anti-inflammatory effects (Ulbricht 2010). It is also used to fight viral infections. Prickly pear has been use by Mexicans for hundreds of years. A study shows that prickly pear cactus can decrease blood sugar levels in people with type 2 diabetes (The Daily Health 2016).

Ginger, the "root" or the rhizome of the plant Zingiber officinale, has been a popular spice and herbal medicine for thousands of years. It has a long tradition of being very effective for digestive system complaints such as upset stomach, diarrhea and nausea and may prevent stomach ulcers (Wolosin & Edelman 2000). Ginger is widely used in Uyghur, Unani, Chinese medicine and Ayurveda as well.

Some studies show that ginger has also been used to help treat arthritis (Ahmet et al. 2005; Wigler 2003). Ginger is a powerful cancer fighter, has anti-inflammatory properties and can provide protection against colorectal and ovarian cancer (Schreiber 2008; Suekawa 1984).

Ginseng is one of the most popular herbs found in North America and in eastern Asia typically in cooler climates. Panax vietnamensis, discovered in Vietnam is the southernmost ginseng known. Ginseng has a lot of health benefits(Wikipedia 2016). According to studies, ginseng shows promise for protecting heart health (Lee & Kim 2014) including anti-hypertensive effects. It is believed to provide an energy boost, lower blood sugar and cholesterol levels, reduce stress, promote relaxation, treat diabetes, and treat sexual dysfunction in men. Many Malaysian Chinese prefer to use to ginseng for various health reasons.

Misai Kucing (Orthosiphon stamineus) known as kidney tea in Malaysia. Misai kucing is a medicinal herb found mainly throughout South East Asia and tropical Australia (Affendy et al. 2011). It has been widely used in Malaysia for treating kidney problems, gout, and diabetes. Studies show that misai kucing has numerous health benefits such as anti-hypertensive, anti-diabetic, cholesterol-inhibiting and tumour-inhibiting effects, as well as relieving of joint and muscle aches (Aziz et al. 2003; Azizan et al. 1996; Khatun et al. 2011).

Sabah Snake Grass (Clinacanthus nutans L.) is another famous herb and is used in cancer prevention, to improve blood circulation, regulate kidney function, detoxification, regulate the cholesterol and blood pressure, originally found and is grown in tropical countries like Malaysia and Thailand. In Malaysia, it is known as Belalai Gajah or Sabah Snake Grass. It is believed to have beneficial effects on patients with cancer (Yong 2013), although it is also used to reduce symptoms attributed to dialysis. Currently, there is not enough evidence on the herb's effectiveness so it is necessary to undertake more research.

This plant is a well-known anti-snake venom amongst the traditional healers of Thailand. Sabah snake grass is utilized in Malaysia as a traditional medicine, particularly for treating skin rashes, scorpion and insect bites. A study showed that the methanolic extract of Sabah snake grass leaves showed significant antibacterial activity against all the tested microorganisms (Arullappan 2014; Sekar 2016). In Indonesia, sabah snake grass is known as dandang gendis and is used locally to treat patients with kidney failure.

Ghasemzadeh et al. (2014) showed that sabah snake grass is a good natural antioxidant. Yoke Keong Yong et al. (2013) also showed that snake grass extracts possess antioxidant and antiproliferative properties against cultured cancer cell lines. A study showed that sabah snake grass is a good natural antioxidant (Arullappan 2014).

Turmeric (Curcuma longa) has been used in Asia for thousands of years. It is commonly used in Indian, Uyghur, Chinese and Malay medicine etc. It grows wild in the forests of South and Southeast Asia. It is one of the key ingredients in many Asian dishes especially Indian dishes and is called the "Queen of Spices". It contains a wide range of antioxidant, antiviral, antibacterial, antifungal, anticarcinogenic, antimutagenic and anti-inflammatory properties (Ramsewak et al. 2000). Many studies showed the health benefits of turmeric. Few studies have proved that it has potential anticancer activity (Kuttan et al. 1985). It showed antiviral activity. Turmeric treats wound, bruises, inflamed joints and sprains. Nozomi Hishikawa et al. (2012) suggested a significant improvement of the behavioral symptoms in Alzheimer's disease with turmeric treatment. It is under study for its potential to affect human diseases, including Alzheimer's disease and diabetes (Mishra & Palanivelu 2008).

Rokok resdung or lilin resdung is a common treatment for sinusitis in Malay traditional medicine. Traditional Malay treatment would treat sinus in a traditional way. Usually it is made of 100% cotton. Face Candling is a simple natural remedy for treating sinusitis with herb candles. The content in rokok resung may vary for example herbs, citronella, sea cucumber and honey. The procedure to use rokok resdung is first to light up the end of rokok resdung. This will cause the other end of it to produce smoke. Spread the smoke evenly along the face. The smell is quite strong and it comes inside the nose canal. It can be a bit hard to bear. Yellowish dust will remain on the face after treatment which is considered as toxic. Wipe carefully the yellowish powder and wash off the face.

Malay postnatal care (Malay confinement) is also very common in Malaysia, Indonesia as well as in Singapore. The purpose of postnatal care is to regain energy and overall recover and take care of the mother's health in later life and it reduces the postnatal depression. Normally, the confinement period is 44 days, but some women continue up to 100 days. Most of the women prefer to use this traditional practice. The postnatal care service can start within the first week of birth if the mother has gone through normal birth. If the mother has experienced caesarean birth, the service starts 14 days after delivery and also only light pressure will be applied to the abdomen.

Postnatal wrap (bengkong) is important part of the postnatal care service after finishing the massage and carried out by the confinement lady or an older experienced women. Around 15 meters long cloth is used for wrapping. It is called postpartum abdominal wrapping or bengkung wrap. Normally, some medicinal herbs and oil are put on the bengkong. Applying hot compression and taking herbal baths are part of this process.

It is believed that applying hot compression is to dissolves residual blood clots in the womb and cleanses the womb. Various herbs are used for preparing the compress.

Postpartum abdominal wrapping (Bengkung Wrap) is a good way to aid postpartum slimming, an important device for quicker recovery after childbirth.

Photo: Postpartum abdominal wrapping
(Binder) or Bengkung Wrap

Herbal steam bath is also helpful for detoxification, to boost, circulation, lifting the womb and to improve the woman's health. However, during the confinement period women avoid consuming cold foods and drinks. But during the pregnancy, many Malay women avoid eating overheated food and prefer to consume cold foods and drinks. Many of the Malay Muslim do pray or make dua during the labor for safety and to control their anxiety. In this case, it is a very powerful meditation. After delivery, the father of the newborn may read the azan into the infant's right ear and iqamah (takbir) into the left ear. It is not only for religious purposes, but also it is beneficial for comforting the babies.

Eating and Drinking (Pantang Makan dan Minum) is also an important part of postnatal care. This refers to the prohibition of eating and drinking certain food items. Generally, Malays believe that cooling foods are not good for the mothers and infants. They believe that cooling foods causes poor circulation. So, avoid eating cucumber, banana, cabbage and cold drinks. Also, acidic foods like lemon, lime and pineapple are not good for the baby. Some women even drink only Jamu. Some mothers who have just delivered take a drink called Jamu (Djamu). Jamu is a famous Indonesian drink. Jamu is believed to keep the body warm.

Chinese, Indian and other minorities have their own postnatal care. Purpose of having Chinese confinement foods is supplying the strengths and revitalizing for new mothers.

3. Traditional Chinese Medicine

Traditional Chinese medicine (TCM) began with the coming of the Chinese migrants. TCM included Chinese herbal medicine, acupuncture and moxibustion, tuinalogy, cupping and Qigong. TCM is used for post stroke, chronic pain such as back and neck pain; knee joint inflammation, sprain of leg/hand, insomnia, depression, hypertension, diabetes, early stage cancer, early stage dementia, cardio-vascular diseases, constipation, indigestion, asthma, cough, and flue.

Acupuncture, Chinese herbal medicine, chiropractic care, traditional Chinese cupping (ba guan), traditional Chinese scraping (gua sha), tuina, moxibustion, qigong, reflexology and herbal footbath therapy have been practiced in Chinese medicine in Malaysia.

There are some TCM practitioner bodies in Malaysia which are registered with the Ministry of Health such as Malaysian Chinese Medical Association (MCMA) which has more than 900 members, Federation of Chinese Physicians and Medicine-Dealers Association of Malaysia (FCPMDAM) which has more than 4000 members and Federation of Chinese Physicians & Acupuncturists Association of Malaysia (FCPAAM). FCPAAM was founded in 2001 and qualified to register in Council for Societies Registration of Malaysia Government. Today, there are more than 3,000 members in the Federation of Chinese Physicians and Acupuncturists Association of Malaysia (FCPAAM).

4. Indian Medicine

Indian medicine includes Ayurveda, Unani medicine, Siddha and Yoga. Indian medicine has been practiced since the 19th century in Malaysia. Ayurveda, One of the world's oldest holistic healthcare systems, has been around for more than 5,000 years (Ragozin 2016). Today it is popular among the Indian community in Malaysia, but Muslims cannot practice Yoga as it is prohibited by the religion (The telegraph 2008).

Ayurveda treatment and wellness centers are dedicated to helping people access deeper levels of contentment, rejuvenation and holistic treatment by qualified Ayurvedic physicians and trained Ayurvedic therapists in Malaysia.

5. Homeopathy

Homeopathy is based on Samuel Hahnemann's doctrine of 'like cures like', according to which a substance that causes the symptoms of a disease in healthy people will cure similar symptoms in sick people. Homeopathic remedies are based on plant, mineral and animal substances. The first Malay known to have practiced homeopathy was Dr. Burhanuddin Al-Helmy (1911-1969) (Globinmed 2015).

However, it is unclear the date of practicing of Homeopathy in Malaysia, many homeopathic practitioners believe that around 1940 homeopathy was introduced by Indians through the British army. The first homeopathic clinic was set up in Johor Bahru (Globinmed 2015).

Cyberjaya University College for Medical Sciences (CUCMS) offers first degree course in homeopathy (BHMS). The Bachelor of Homeopathic Medical Science (Hons) is the first and only programme in homeopathy in Malaysia in CUCMS. It is designed with an integrated approach towards education and health. This programme is in line with the Ministry of Health's efforts to gradually integrate T&CM into the government and private healthcare sectors. Homeopathy continues to gain acceptance in Malaysia (Cyberjaya University College for Medical Sciences 2015).

6. Complementary Medicine

Complementary Medicine includes Chiropractor, naturopathy, nutritional therapy, osteopathy, hypnotherapy, aromatherapy, Spa therapy, reflexology, therapeutic massage, Thai, Balinese,

Javanese, Swedish, Shiatsu massage, psychotherapy, colour vibration therapy, crystal healing, aura metaphysic, ozone therapy, chelation therapy and reiki etc. Complementary Medicine is divided as:

Mind-body and soul therapy: Mind-body and soul therapy focuses on the interactions among the brain, mind, body and behavior, and on the powerful ways in which emotional, social, spiritual, mental and behavioral factors can directly affect health such as meditation, hypnotherapy, prayer for health reasons and psychotherapy etc.

Biological-based practices: It is one of the major areas of complementary medicine. The complementary medicine domain of biologically based practices includes, but is not limited to, botanicals, animal-derived extracts, vitamins, minerals, fatty acids, amino acids, proteins, prebiotics and probiotics, whole diets, and functional foods which is including nutritional therapy, naturopathy, ozone therapy and chelation therapy.

Manipulative and body-based practices: it focuses on the structures and systems of the body such as chiropractic, osteopathy, therapeutic massage, Shiatsu, Swedish, Thai, Balinese/Javanese massage, midwifery, cupping therapy and reflexology.

Energy medicine: Energy medicine deals with energy fields such as colour vibration therapy, phytobiophysics, aura metaphysics, crystal healing, bach flower remedy, roaha and reiki etc.

Malay massage, acupuncture, herbal medicine and Malay postnatal care are most commonly practiced in T&CM integrated hospitals in Malaysia.

CURRENT STATUS OF TRADITIONAL AND COMPLEMENTARY MEDICINE IN MALAYSIA

T&CM, which includes herbal medicine, has become increasingly popular in its worldwide application including Malaysia. From 2000 to 2005, annual sales for traditional medicines increased from USD 385 million (RM 1 billion) to USD 1.29 billion (RM 4.5 billion) (Abuduli 2015).

The prevalence and factors associated with its use are largely unknown, although the use is believed to be widespread. The Malaysian government has been encouraging all the initiatives and researches on this particular field in recent years. The MOH has taken a positive and proactive approach towards T&CM, as well as herbal medicine by implementing various measures to ensure quality, safety for the consumers and maintaining its healthy development.

There are 12 modalities in the diploma and degree in T&CM curriculum in Malaysia; they are Malay massage, natural medicine, reflexology, homoeopathy, chiropractic, acupuncture, aromatherapy, TCM, Malay medicine, Ayurvedic medicine and Islamic medicine. There are six universities and colleges offering T&CM courses. Currently, there are 6 different T&CM practices provided which include:

PRACTICE OF TRADITIONAL AND COMPLEMENTARY MEDICINE AMONG HEALTH PROFESSIONALS IN MALAYSIA

1) Traditional Malay massage for chronic pain and post stroke management
2) Acupuncture for chronic pain, anaesthesia and post stroke management
3) Herbal therapy as an adjunct treatment for cancer
4) Malay postnatal care
5) Shirodhara (it is a form of Ayurveda therapy)
6) External Basti Therapy

Traditional Malay massage and acupuncture are used for chronic pain and stroke; herbal oncology is used for complement treatment with allopathy therapy; and postnatal massage is used to relieve muscle cramps and fatigues after labour. Shirodhara is used for insomnia, headache, stress or mental fatigue, anxiety & mild depression. External basti therapy is unique and effective for musculoskeletal treatment (Vinjamury et al. 2014).

Massage has been practiced for thousands of years. Today, if you need or want a massage, you can choose from among 80 types of massage therapies with a wide variety of pressures, movements, and techniques. These all involve pressing, rubbing, or manipulating muscles and other soft tissues with hands and fingers, sometimes even forearms, elbows, or feet are used.

"Massage" means the manipulation of the soft tissues of the human body with the hand, foot, arm or elbow, whether or not such manipulation is aided by hydrotherapy, thermal therapy any electrical or mechanical device or the application to the human body of a chemical or herbal preparation.

Massage is "urut" in Malay language. Traditional Malay massage is based on the kampung massage practice. There are many kinds of massage and Malay massage makes extensive use of the different types of herbal oils. This comprehensive and effective massage therapy helps to relax the nerves and mind. The Malay massage is a mixture of kneading, stroking and pressing with hands.

Malay massage is divided into two types based on their purpose; wellness and therapeutic massage. For the purpose of wellness, the massage helps in reducing anxiety, improving sleep, boosting immunity of the body and reducing stress. Massage has three categories, namely relaxation massage, rejuvenating massage and improving blood circulation massage. Therapeutic massage helps to improve the condition of a particular illness and in reducing severity of pain especially for sprains and low back pain. Therapeutic massages are specified into massage of nerve ailments, joint ailments, sprains, muscle ailments and others.

Treatment massage takes a variety of forms and may last between 15-90 minutes. Many patients with chronic pain and post stroke get treatment massage and satisfied from T&CM department so far. Treatment massage takes 15-45 minutes for chronic pain and 60-90 minutes for post stroke case. Massage is administered as a complement to other therapy, medical or rehabilitation therapy and in some cases it is only carried out with the approval of a medical practitioner. The general benefits of massage are to relieve stress, encourage relaxation, help manage pain, relax muscles and improve flexibility and range of motion.

Acupuncture is one of the main modalities of treatment in traditional Chinese medicine and can be traced back more than 2000 years in China (Liu et al. 2013). It mainly involves the theory of meridians, location, usage, indications of acupoints and needling manipulations. Acupuncture can be performed manually (manual acupuncture) or electrically (electric acupuncture). Needle acupuncture treatment is effective for postoperative and chemotherapy nausea and vomiting, nausea of pregnancy, and post-operative dental pain. It is also effective as an adjust therapy in stroke rehabilitation, headache, menstrual cramps, tennis elbow, fibromyalgia (general muscle pain), low back pain, carpal-tunnel syndrome and asthma.

Acupuncture is particularly useful in resolving physical problem-related tension, stress and emotional conditions. Acupuncture treatment can be given at the same time with other medicine such as conventional western medicine. Acupuncture has been well accepted by Chinese patients and is widely used to improve motor, sensation, speech and other neurological functions in patients with stroke since it is a relatively simple, inexpensive and safe treatment compared to other conventional interventions.

Many studies involving thousands of patients have been published and they indicate that patients get well faster, perform better in self-care, require less nursing and rehabilitation therapy and cost less in terms of healthcare expenditure after being treated with acupuncture post-stroke. Back pain is among the most prevalent health complaints of mankind. It has been estimated that up to 80% of the world's population will suffer from back pain at some point in their lives with the lower back being the most common location of pain (American Chiropractic Association 2008). Back pain is also the most frequent indication for using unconventional therapies. Survey data suggests that back pain is one of the most common indications for referral to acupuncturists. Many people who have chronic low back pain have found acupuncture to be helpful.

Herbal therapy is provided for the purpose of improving quality of life, boosting body immunity, reducing side effects of chemotherapy and radiotherapy and synergistic effect of anti-cancer drugs (Liao et al. 2013). In Malaysia, malignant neoplasm persisted as one of the five principal causes of national mortality (Ministry of Health Malaysia 2009). In 2005, cancer contributed to more than 10% of all deaths in government hospitals (Subramaniam 2013). The aims of herbal therapy are to reduce side effects of cancer treatment, improve body immune system and synergistic effect. Herbal therapy used for adjusting cancer treatment will focus on six types of the most prevalent cancers in Malaysia; they are breast, lung, cervix, nasopharynx, colorectal and liver (Dhanoa 2014).

The prevalence of herb use ranges from 60 to 80% among cancer patients depending on the definition of herbal medicine used in each study, sample size, and the place where the study was conducted. A population-based survey indicated that about a quarter of cancer patients had consulted an herbal medicine practitioner in the past in UK (Tavakoli et al. 2012). A Canadian study shows that 20% of breast cancer patients used at least one herbal medicine treatment in the past (Gray et al. 2003) whereas American studies more consistently report rates well above 65%, such rates are considerably higher than those reported in general population or among other cancer diagnostic groups (Creek et al. 1998; Morris et al. 2009)

Several herbs have been shown to have different effects on immune effector cells and cytokine levels in laboratory, animal and human studies (Amirghofran 2012). This is manifested as impaired humoral and cell-mediated responsiveness as well as decreased nonspecific defense mechanisms. All cancer patients seeking for adjunct treatment at Traditional and Complementary Medicine (T&CM) Unit in Malaysia should be referred by a medical oncologist, properly investigated and a precise diagnosis must have been made in Malaysia.

The following herbs have shown to have different effects on immune effecter cells and cytokine levels in laboratories, animal and human studies:

Radix astragali (huang qi), radix salviae miltiorrhizae (dan shen), rhizoma atra ct ylodis macrocephalae (bai zhu), fructus ligustri lucidi (nu zhen zi), radix salix (liu zhi), fructus lycii chinensis (gao qi zi), fructus ligustri lucidi (nu zhen zi), radix ginseng (ren shen), radix et caulis jixueteng (ji xue teng) and radix angelicae sinensis (dang gui) etc (Cohen et al; Ministry of Health 2009).

Malay postnatal care is used to prevent "meroyan" (postnatal depression) as this complication may arise in postnatal period. The incidence of postnatal depression is low in Malaysia (estimated to be 3.9%) due to vast majority of Malaysian women still believing in the traditional postnatal beliefs and practices (MOH 2005). Malay postpartum period is called confinement period. There are three major features in Malay postnatal care; using herbs, heat and Malay postnatal massage. The T&CM unit will implement the manipulative component of Malay postnatal care. The services consist of wellness postnatal massage and midwifery care.

Malays postpartum period is called "masa dalam pantang". The literal translation means "confinement period". Traditionally, a woman remains at home during this period. During this time, her behaviour in relation to diet, activity and hygiene is determined by tradition, and the theory behind traditional Malay medicine which underlies some of these beliefs and practices. The behaviour around diet, activity and hygiene that comprises the "confinement period" is to restore her energy and health after childbirth.

There are four major features in Malay postnatal care: Postnatal care of neonatal, diet and confinement for postpartum mother, the use of herbs, Malay postnatal massage. Malay Postnatal massage includes whole body massage, hot compression (bertungku) and body wrapping (barut). Body massage is done at least six to seven times during the confinement period.

Herbal preparations, acupuncture and traditional massage are the three elements which would be introduced in the hospitals conducting the pilot projects (Abuduli 2011).

TRADITIONAL AND COMPLEMENTARY MEDICINE INTEGRATED HOSPITALS

There are total of 14 hospitals where T&CM practices are integrated into the modern healthcare system to achieve a holistic approach towards enhancing health and quality of life since 2015.

Traditional Malay Massage is available in Kelapa Batus Hospital in Pulau Pinang, Hospital Putrajaya in W.P. Putrajaya, Hospital Sultan Ismail in Johor Bharu, Hospital Duchess of Kent in Sabah, Hospital Sultanah Nur Zahirah in Kuala Terengganu, Sarawak General Hospital in Kuching, Hospital Port Dickson in Seremban, Hospital Sultanah Bahiyah in Alor Setar, Sultanah Hajjah Kalsom Hospital in Kameron Highlands, Raja Perempuan Zainab II Hospital in Kota Bharu, Kelantan, Cheras Rehabilitation Hospital, Sabah Woman and Children Hospital and Jasin Hospital in Melaka. Acupuncture is not only integrated above 13 hospitals but also in National Cancer Institute.

Traditional postnatal care is practiced in Hospital Kelapa Batus, Hospital Putrajaya, Hospital Sultan Ismail, Hospital Duchess of Kent, Hospital Sultanah Nur Zahirah, Hospital Sultanah Bahiyah, Sarawak General Hospital, Raja Perempuan Zainab II Hospital, Jasin Hospital and 1 Malaysia Low Risk Birth Center MAIW.

National Center Institute, Hospital Sultan Ismail, Hospital Kelapa Batus and Sabah Woman and Children Hospital practiced herbal therapy as an adjust treatment for cancer.

Shirodhara and external basti therapy is practiced in Cheras Rehabilitation Hospital and Hospital Port Dickson.

TRADITIONAL AND COMPLEMENTARY MEDICINE OVERVIEW AND ITS IMPORTANCE IN MALAYSIA

T&CM has played an important role in public health not only in Malaysia but also all over the world. For the past few decades, traditional medicine has made significant contributions to the health care of Malaysian people and it is widely acknowledged that the practices and applications of herbal medicine are widespread and increasing at a progressive pace in Malaysia. Malaysia's rich tropical biodiversity is a reliable source of natural health products. In order to take full advantage of natural resources, research and development (R&D) on Malaysian herb has become of prime interest in most universities and research institutions (Editorial Committee Traditional and Complementary Medicine Division 2011).

The Malaysian government has given substantial support and since 1985, specific research funding has been allocated through its Intensified Research in Priority Areas (IRPA) programme (Jamal 2006).

In 1999, sales of herbal products worldwide had been aggregated to USD80 billion (RM 279 billion). The Malaysian market for herbal or natural products medicinal plant and aromatic plants including aquatic animals is estimated at RM4.6 billion with an annual growth projection of 15 to 20

per cent (Jamal 2006; Burke et al. 2006). More Malaysians will seek the T&CM services in the future. (Mohd Zin 2009).

In Malaysia, the market for traditional medicine was estimated at RM2.6 billion (US$0.84 billion) in 2007, and is expected to reach USD156 billion (RM483.61 billion) in 2050 based on annual growth rate of 10 percent (Akademi Sains Malaysia 2011). In the near future, we will be witnessing integration of T&CM and it shall be an important component of the prime healthcare system worldwide. It will co-exist with modern medicine and contribute towards enhancing the health and quality of life of all Malaysians.

Since there has been no formal education or training on T&CM provided for western trained health professionals, it is crucial to have a clear understanding on the practice of T&CM. Carrying out a research on current applications and practices of T&CM in Malaysia along with the knowledge and attitude to be associated with practice is not only highly imperative in terms of identifying current progress, existing challenges to be addressed, but also significantly important in providing valuable information for government bodies to come out with efficient and facilitative strategies, supportive measurements and guidelines for further development of T&CM in Malaysia (Shih et al. 2008).

POTENTIAL BENEFITS OF THIS STUDY

This study will help to provide the following benefits:

1. The outcome of the study will help to provide accurate and up-to-date information with regards to T&CM.

2. The results from this study can help us know more information about the practice, knowledge, and attitude towards T&CM.
3. The study can attract the attention of people on T&CM.
4. The study can attract the attention of International Organizations about T&CM.
5. The study can help further development in making decisions about integration of T&CM into mainstream medicine.

GENERAL ISSUES

As unavoidable consequence of almost a century of absolute predominance of Western Medicine (WM)/Conventional Medicine (CM) across the world driven by phenomenal breakthroughs in all disciplines of natural sciences, T&CM has been inadvertently dispelled from mainstream healthcare system, overlooked in value, even prohibited in certain countries by legal decrees (Shih et al. 2003).

However, due to the fact that a large part of the population in developing countries still rely on traditional practitioners and local medicinal plants to satisfy their primary health care needs (in some Asian and African countries, 80% of the population depend on traditional medicine for primary health care) (WHO 2003) plus the high cost of health insurance, population ageing and other reasons have propelled the public to seek other types of T&CM in many developed countries. Fueled by this urgent and pressing demand, T&CM has been

PRACTICE OF TRADITIONAL AND COMPLEMENTARY MEDICINE AMONG HEALTH PROFESSIONALS IN MALAYSIA

gaining a new momentum in most of the countries since the last decade.

The popularity and demand for medicinal plants as health supplements or for medical purposes have been increasing worldwide. The increasing use of T&CM including herbal medicines by the Malaysian public is of special concern especially because T&CM products are not rigorously regulated by the Drug Control Authority (DCA) of Malaysia.

Currently, there is lack of regulatory and legal mechanism, inadequate evidence, lack of formulized training and lack of public information regarding the rational use of T&CM. Future strategic direction for T&CM in Malaysia concerns the area of practitioners training, regulation and international collaboration and research specifically patient satisfaction and quality of life and service offered (WHO 2010).

RESEARCH QUESTIONS

1. Is practice on T&CM high among health professionals?
2. What factors are associated with practice on T&CM among health professionals?
3. Is there any association between knowledge and attitude regarding T&CM and T&CM usage among health professionals?
4. Which modalities of T&CM are most practiced among health professionals?

RESEARCH JUSTIFICATION

There are substantial numbers of published studies related to knowledge, attitude and practice (KAP) of T&CM among western-trained doctors, students, patients, especially elderly and adults in other countries, which were mostly conducted in western developed countries.

In many parts of the world, health professionals may neglect the applications of T&CM in their clinical practices or their knowledge and requisite attitude on T&CM and its practice may not be adequate. There has been no research so far carried out to investigate the practice about T&CM among health professionals in Malaysia. This prompted the researcher to conduct a study on this topic in an attempt of promoting and facilitating the T&CM practices and research in this country. It would ensure a bright future for T&CM in Malaysia if more and constant efforts are made to contribute to this field. This study also could be another attempt on the above endeavor in further development of T&CM research in Malaysia. T&CM is garnering increasing interest and acceptance among the general population.

Although T&CM applications are thought to be popular among Malaysian population, studies about practices on T&CM among the health professionals have not been done in Malaysia. Health professionals' knowledge, practical experiences and requisite attitude are mandatory to facilitate applications of T&CM and educate the patients alike. Therefore, the purpose of this study is to measure the practice on T&CM among health professionals and to explore factors associated with T&CM application.

Although the Malaysian Government-Ministry of Health has been encouraging the practice of T&CM, patients/clients would not be able to apply it for their need of medical treatments or sometimes it leads to negative outcomes due to lack of knowledge on T&CM and its safe applications. T&CM is chosen as the topic of interest because T&CM is commonly practiced and frequently spotlighted as a key area where health professionals' practice, knowledge and requisite attitude reflect a serious inadequacy. Most of the western-trained physicians are ignorant of the benefits and risks of T&CM.

The popularity of T&CM and their increasing clinical significance were the driving force for initiating this study. Due to ever increasing popularity of natural health products consumption in Malaysia, the health professionals' role with respect to natural health products is important to consider. As health professionals, it has been argued that physicians should be able to provide information about all the T&CM products. It is the health professionals' responsibility to improve the safety of medication by monitoring and preventing adverse interactions including the risks posed by herb-drug interactions.

Although T&CM as well as herbal products are natural and have less side effects comparatively, sometimes it causes more dangerous health problems or it influences treatment in its miss-applications. In the view of the critical roles that could be played by medical professionals as information providers to their patients in terms of safety and efficacy of T&CM and western medicine (WM)-T&CM interactions, health professionals have a leading role to play in integrating T&CM into the mainstream medicine. Therefore, it is of paramount importance to identify the current practice of T&CM among health professionals and evaluate the feasibility of capacitating health professionals in consulting their patients on traditional and complementary treatments by offering re-education and training in T&CM.

OBJECTIVES

1. General Objective

To determine the practice of T&CM and factors associated with it among the health professionals in five selected hospitals in Malaysia.

2. Specific Objectives

1. To determine the rate of T&CM usage among health professionals.
2. To identify the type of T&CM modalities used by the health professionals.
3. To determine the association between socio-demographic factors and T&CM usage among the health professionals.
4. To determine the association between knowledge regarding T&CM and T&CM usage among the health professionals.

5. To determine the association between attitude regarding T&CM and T&CM usage among the health professionals.
6. To determine the association between reasons of using T&CM and T&CM usage among the health professionals.
7. To determine the association between education/training in T&CM and T&CM usage among the health professionals.

REASEACH HYPOTHESES

1. Rate of practicing T&CM is higher among doctors than nurses and pharmacists.
2. The most commonly used T&CM modalities are massage and herbal medicine.
3. Malay, female, Muslim, well-educated, wealthy and senior health professionals practiced T&CM more than others.
4. Level of knowledge is higher among T&CM user than non-user.
5. Level of positive attitude is higher among T&CM user than non-user.
6. The main reason of using T&CM is to maintain health.
7. Health education and training influences the practice of T&CM.

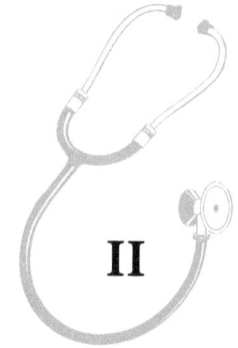

II

LITERATURE REVIEW

THE PRACTICE OF TRADITIONAL AND COMPLEMENTARY MEDICINE

The Practice of T&CM by Health Professionals

In Birmingham Heartlands Hospital, 30% of the doctors had personally used CAMs and 56.0% of their families had used CAMs (Fountain-Polley 2007). In one study, majority of the pediatricians would consider using CAM for themselves, but only 37.2% have used some of the CAM therapies listed. Relaxation, massage therapy, prayer healing, and herbs were the most commonly used therapies. In another study, 10.3% of the pediatricians used T&CM (**Sawni &Thomas 2007**). Xu & Levine (2008) showed that 38.0% of the medical residents had never personally used herbal medicine, while 46.0% had previously used a product. A study in Israel found that 87.3% nurses and midwives used CAM (Samuels et al. 2010).

PRACTICE OF TRADITIONAL AND COMPLEMENTARY MEDICINE AMONG HEALTH PROFESSIONALS IN MALAYSIA

The Practice of T&CM by Patients

The number of patients seeking alternative and herbal therapy is growing exponentially (Pal & Shukla 2003). Half of 26 medical residents and clinical clerks estimated that between 11-30% of their patients were using herbal medicines; none of the respondents estimated more than 70.0% of their patients were using herbal medicines. Twenty of 25 medical residents and clinical clerks believed that less than 10% of their patients could use herbal medicines safely (Xu & Levine 2008). A cross-sectional study conducted on knowledge, attitudes and practice on complementary and alternative medicine (CAM) among general practitioners in Doha, Qatar found that 30.1% had practiced it, 24.8% referred patients and 34.8% general practitioners asked the patients about whether they use CAM (Al Shaar et al. 2010).

A total of 69.4% of the Malaysians have been using T&CM in their whole life and 55.6% of the population used it at least in 12 months period (WHO 2010). This could well be gross under-reporting, as studies around the world have shown that more than 40% of the population in many countries are using T&CM for their healthcare needs (MOH 2004). A study conducted in Taiwan by Yeh et al. (2000) who interviewed 63 primary caregivers discovered a CAM usage prevalence rate of 73% (Lim et al. 2006).

According to the Natural Health Products Directorate (NHPD) of Canada, 71% of Canadians have taken at least a natural health product such as herbal remedies (Johnson et al. 2008). A recent national survey reported that four out of every ten Americans used at least one form of CAM, and one out of five used prescription medications together with CAM (Chagan et al. 2005). A study showed that 26 of the 49 CAM users (53.1%) had used one or more forms of CAM since birth (Lim et al. 2006).

A study showed that more than half (58%) of the general practitioners (GPs) reported recommending CAM to their patients in Italy (Giannelli et al. 2007). A study carried out in Bursa province, Turkey showed that only 29% of GPs were using some types of CAM for themselves (Ozcakir et al. 2007).

Modalities

A survey was carried out on attitude and patterns of CAM usage by German physicians and the findings revealed that the methods most prescribed were physical therapies (71%), phytomedicines (67%), exercises (63%), nutritions and dietings (62%), massages (61%), relaxation techniques (55%), followed by more typical CAM interventions such as homeopathy (38%), acupuncture (37%), and traditional Chinese medicine (18%) (Stange et al. 2008). In Shenyang (China), it was reported that among the western-trained doctors using TCM, 90.6% used herbal remedies, 32.4% used acupuncture and 5.8% used massage in 2001 (Harmworth & Lewith 2001).

Among all CAM therapies, 67.1%, 48.6%, 42.2%, 40.5% and 39.9% nurse-midwives in Israel used massage, herbal medicine, meditation, touch therapies and prayer respectively (Samuels et al. 2010). Another study showed that acupuncture was more frequently recommended than chiropractic and massage (Sewitch et al. 2008).

PRACTICE OF TRADITIONAL AND COMPLEMENTARY MEDICINE AMONG HEALTH PROFESSIONALS IN MALAYSIA

Around two-third of GPs (69.2%) recommended acupuncture, almost half of the GPs (47.9%) recommended manipulative therapy and one-third (38.1%) recommended homeopathy in Tuscany, Italy (Giannelli et al. 2007). A study showed that most of GPs (80.4%) had been practicing CAM and almost one-third of the GPs (29%) were using some types of CAM for themselves and more than one third of GPs (39.2%) used herbs in 2004 in Turkey (Ozcakir et al. 2007).

In a study, the therapies most commonly used in their personal remedy for themselves or family were: massage therapies (34%), acupuncture/acupressure and aromatherapy (20.5%) and herbs and megavitamins (17%). Therapies that were most commonly referred were massage (39%) and acupuncture/acupressure (34%) in the US (Sawni & Thomas 2007).

The Influence of Socio-Demographic Factors

A study showed that T&CM use was associated with gender, age, race, marital status, income level and health status. The odds of women to be in a category of "using herbal medicines" were 1.8 times higher than that of men, in which those with health problems were 2.3 times higher compared to those without health problems (Aziz & Tey 2009). According to a survey in primary care clinic in Kuching, Sarawak, Malaysia from January to April 2004, 51.4% patients used CAM and 47.8% of those patients used more than one type of CAM. Utilization rates of CAM were found to be associated with employment status but not with other socio-demographic factors (Lee et al. 2007). About 30% of surgeons regularly utilized TCM in their clinical practice, often to enhance recovery from surgical intervention (Harmworth & Lewith 2001). Sewitch et al. (2008) found that physicians were more negative compared to than other health care professionals. Younger physicians were more likely to recommend CAM compared with their senior colleagues and who had more working experience.

Knowledge Regarding T&CM

Canadian pharmacists themselves have identified their lack of knowledge about natural health products, especially in the areas of mechanisms of action, adverse effects, drug interactions, and dosage (Johnson et al. 2008). In one study, 85% of those surveyed agreed that knowledge about CAM would play an important role in their future as practicing physicians. The results of this study agreed with the previous statements as the first-and-second-year students have similar belief towards CAM (Riccard & Skelton 2008).

There was a clear consensus that TCM (mainly herbal medicine) was useful and safe in treating patients with chronic or intractable illnesses (Harmworth & Lewith 2001). A research conducted in Japan in 1999 and 2005 indicated that Kampo **was most commonly known to doctors (72%) in 1999 and 83% in 2005.** The doctors who possessed knowledge of CAM including herbal therapy increased significantly from 1999 to 2005 (Fujiwara et al. 2011). A substantial proportion of pediatric cancer patients utilized CAM therapies, often without their physician's knowledge (Lim et al. 2006). In Turkey GPs knowledge levels in CAM were low (60.8%). About half of them (51%) believed in the efficiency of CAM.

GPs desired more information about herbal medicine and acupuncture (Ozcakir et al. 2007).

Attitude Towards T&CM

Older and better qualified doctors clearly had stronger positive feelings about TCM than younger doctors (Harmworth & Lewith 2001). In the near future, 58% of doctors desired to practice CAM therapies. Previous survey demonstrated that although the term 'CAM' was recognized by only 45% of medical doctors, CAM were practiced by 73% doctors, and the most common CAM practiced was Kampo (Fujiwara et al. 2011). The majority of Israelis nurse-midwives were using and recommending CAM to their patients and believed that CAM can complement conventional medical therapies. Pediatricians have a positive attitude towards CAM (Sawni & Thomas 2007). A study said that positive attitude towards CAM did not correlate with CAM referrals (Sewitch et al. 2008).

Education and Training in T&CM

A study on attitude towards traditional Chinese medicine (TCM) among the western trained doctors in Shenyang, Northern China, showed that 98% of respondents had some theoretical and practical TCM training; 15% had additional postgraduate training; the older doctors had more training than their recently qualified colleagues and older doctors used their training more, 35% used it weekly and 15% used it daily. The length of TCM training in university varied widely amongst western trained doctors. Training was longer and more detail for older doctors (Harmworth & Lewith 2001).

The vast majority of physicians (96.5%) reported that they had not received any education about CAM modalities. Although more than half of the GPs (62.7%) agreed with the necessity for CAM education, the knowledge levels about CAM modalities were low, with most physicians (74.4 %) wanting to learn more about CAM in Bursa province, Turkey (Ozcakir et al. 2007).

A study carried out among senior medical students in Israel revealed that 79% of the senior medical students were interested in studying CAM in medical school, and 65% were interested in applying these techniques to treat patients. About 87% of students were familiar with some techniques of complementary medicine (Oberbaum et al. 2003), whereas more than 70% of the doctors in Japan who were trained under the western medical system prescribed Kampo extraction (Oguamanam 2008). A study showed that the use of western medicine and traditional Chinese medicine were significantly associated with the training background of the doctors (Huang et al. 2009). Overall, 86% of physicians and 74% of medical school students felt that complementary medicine education should be incorporated into the medical school curriculum (Xu & Levine 2008). Practicing physicians also seem to be increasingly interested in CAM (Milden & Stokols 2004). In 2002 and 2004, 60% and 81% of the physicians in the U.S. expressed interest in learning more about CAM (Winslow & Shapiro 2002).

Europe report that 10–80% of physicians expressed an interest in CAM, want more education on CAM, have a positive attitude towards CAM, and consider referring patients for CAM but only 18% had any formal training and most of the training was self-taught or Continuous Medical Education (CME) (55%). The majority (84%) of the respondents want more CME courses on CAM, report that CAM modalities should be taught in medical schools (80%) and almost half (49%) reported personal use of CAM therapies (Sawni & Thomas 2007). Milden & Stokols (2004) and Winslow & Shapiro (2002) revealed that 60% and 80% physicians expressed interest in learning more about CAM in the US.

Reasons for Using Traditional and Complementary Medicine

The overall satisfaction with both CAM (76.5% satisfied, 17.6% very satisfied) and conventional treatment (61% satisfied, 27.1% very satisfied) was high. General perception of the parents towards CAM and mainstream medicine were also investigated in the survey. Sixty percent of 73 paediatric cancer patients's parents felt that, as compared to conventional medicine, CAM was more easily obtainable and had fewer side effects. Despite the high prevalence of CAM usage among studied population, only 6% felt it was more effective than conventional medicine. CAM was not deemed to be necessarily safer or cheaper compared to conventional medicine (Lim et al. 2006).

People turn to traditional medicine mainly because it is affordable, readily available, cheap and philosophically compatible with indigenous cultures (UNESCO 2010). More than one-third (42%) of Tuscan (Italy) GPs never recommended CAM, principally for the insufficient evidence of its effectiveness. Among physicians reporting never recommend CAM to patients, about two thirds were not convinced of its effectiveness while approximately one third felt they have not had enough knowledge to be able to recommend it in Tuscany, Italy (Giannelli et al. 2007).

Sewitch et al. (2008) indicated that most significant barriers for not using CAM were lack of evidence for effectiveness, potential side effects and interactions with allopathic treatments. On the other hand, Ozcakir et al. (2007) showed that more than half of the GPs (51.4%) believed in the efficiency of CAM.

Exposure to Practice of T&CM

Information used in choosing CAM therapies was obtained from a wide variety of sources. Most (70.0%) out of 73 patients had more than one source, the most common being friends (51.0%), followed by other patients (32.7%) or parent's knowledge base (self-referral). Two parents (4.0%) identified that the physician or hospital staff as the source of referral to CAM. Eight percent reported using recommendations from the staff of health food stores, but none sought information from CAM practitioners. Interestingly, before cancer diagnosis, parents turned most often to family (44.4%), their own knowledge base (29.6%) and friends (22.2%) for information about CAM (Lim et al. 2006).

Overall, these sources included family or friends (66.1%), medical doctors (56.1%), magazines or books (34.6%), and radio or television or newspapers (22.6%); only 11.3% named the internet as a source (Herman et al. 2006).

CONCEPTUAL FRAMEWORK

The study is centered on five selected government-owned hospitals in both West and East Malaysia to establish the extent of acceptance of the practice of Traditional & Complementary Medicine (T&CM) among the health professionals. Except for UKMMC, each of the other four hospitals has its own separate T&CM unit and for the purpose of this study, is classified as a T&CM-integrated hospital. These four integrated hospitals have facilities to provide a range of T&CM treatments to patients. There are mainly four common modalities of T&CM being catered for in the government-owned hospitals such as massage, acupuncture, herbal medicine and postnatal care under supervision of the Ministry of Health (MOH) of Malaysia.

An understanding of the practice of T&CM among the health professionals and the related factors affecting it are very important to the study. Factors such as knowledge regarding T&CM, attitude towards T&CM, education and training in T&CM, and socio-demographic characteristics of health professionals are very much related to the practice of T&CM. An exposure to T&CM and reasons for using T&CM either due to health-related or non-health-related reasons also play important roles in assessing the practice of T&CM.

Figure 2.1 shows the various factors affecting or influencing the practice of T&CM in the domestic scene

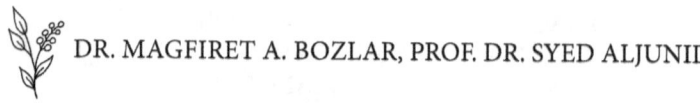

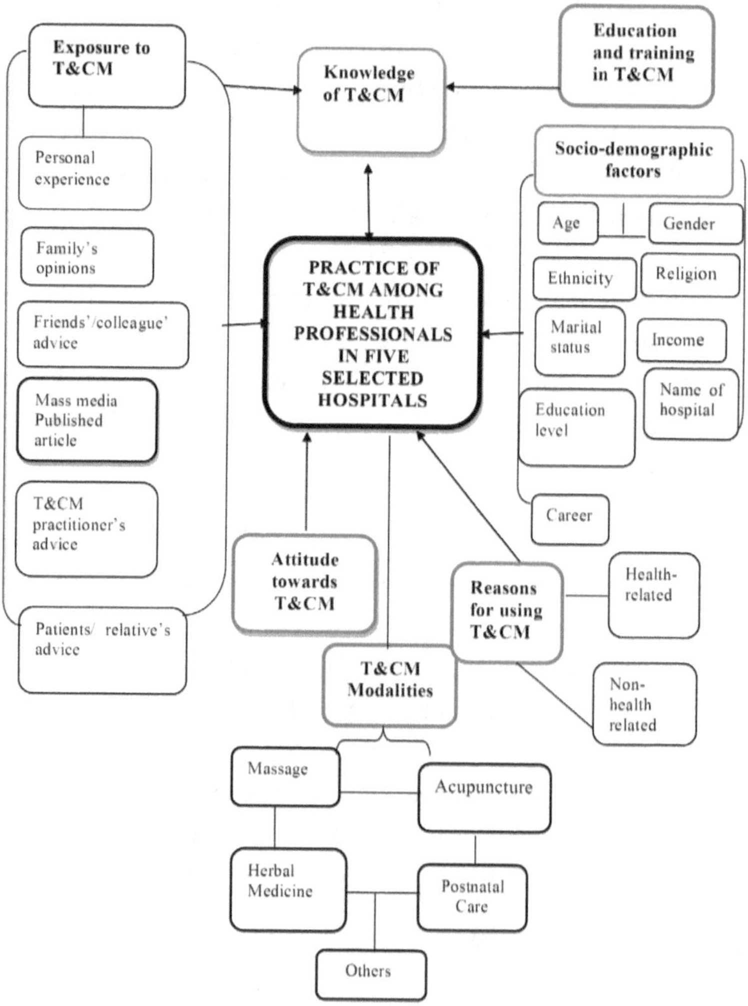

Figure 2.1 Conceptual Framework

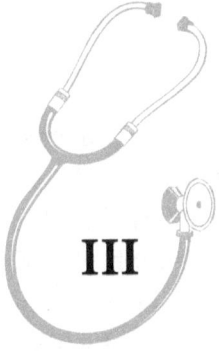

III

METHODOLOGY

INTRODUCTION

This chapter describes the methodology of this study including background of the study location, study design, sampling methods, sample size, study instruments, data collection and analysis and operational definition of variables.

BACKGROUND OF THE STUDY LOCATION

Malaysia is a federal constitutional monarchy in Southeast Asia. It consists of thirteen states and three federal territories and has a total landmass of 330,803 square kilometres separated by the South China Sea into two similarly-sized regions, Peninsular Malaysia (or West Malaysia) and Malaysian Borneo (or East Malaysia) respectively (Malaysia 2016). The capital city is Kuala Lumpur, while Putrajaya is the seat of the federal government. In 2016 the population has exceeded 31,241,000 with over 25 million living on the Peninsular (Peninsular Malaysia 2016).

This study was carried out in Universiti Kebangsaan Malaysia Medical Center (UKMMC), Hospital Putrajaya (HPJ), Hospital Duchess of Kent (HDOK), Sarawak General Hospital (SGH) and Hospital Sultanah Nur Zahirah (HSNZ) which are the main government hospitals in Malaysia. Among the five hospitals, UKMMC is not a T&CM integrated hospital but the other four hospitals are T&CM integrated hospitals. UKMMC, Putrajaya Hospital and Sultanah Nur Zahirah Hospital are situated in West Malaysia whilst Duchess of Kent Hospital and Sarawak General Hospital are situated in East Malaysia as shown in figure 3.1.

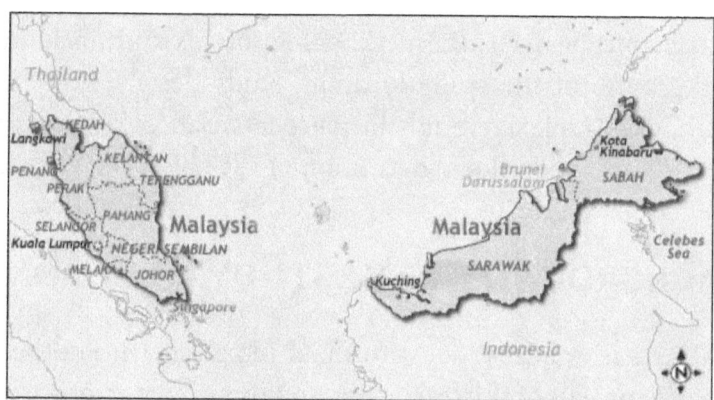

Figure 3.1 Map of Malaysia
Source: MalaysiaMap.org

PRACTICE OF TRADITIONAL AND COMPLEMENTARY MEDICINE AMONG HEALTH PROFESSIONALS IN MALAYSIA

STUDY DESIGN

The design of the study was cross-sectional. The study was carried out using both quantitative and qualitative methods.

STUDY LOCATIONS AND POPULATION

This study was conducted at UKMMC, HPJ, HSNZ, HDOK and SGH (HUS) which are all government hospitals in Malaysia. Except for UKMMC, the other hospitals do provide the T&CM service for the patients. The services provided are mainly traditional Malay massage, acupuncture, herbal medicine and Malay postnatal care.

The population of this study was 500 health professionals (doctors, pharmacists and nurses) who are currently working in five selected hospitals. A total of 100 health professionals were selected from each hospital.

SAMPLING FRAME

The sampling frame was a list of health professionals who are currently working in the five selected hospitals.

SAMPLING UNIT

The sampling unit was each individual health professionals who is currently working in the five selected hospitals in Malaysia.

SAMPLING METHOD

Since the anticipated sample size required for the entire study was to be 500 respondents, 100 respondents were selected randomly from each hospital by using a systematic random sampling according to the staff list in each hospital where a total of 477 questions were collected.

SAMPLE SIZE

The sample size is calculated using the following formula: (Lazereto 2011).

$$n = Z^2 (p\,q) / d^2$$

Calculation of the sample size is based on a rate of 30.1% as the prevalence of practicing T&CM among general practitioners as per the literature review where n is the desired sample size, Z= certainty (for 95%, use 1.96), p (estimated prevalence) = probability of achieving the studied phenomenon; p = 30.1% (0.301), q = (1-p) = complement of the estimated prevalence q = 1- p which is 0.699 and d = (desired precision) = margin of error d = 0.05 (Damião, 2002).

$$n = \frac{1.96^2\,(0.301)*(1-0.301)}{(0.05)^2}$$

N = 323
N + 30% non-response rate
323*30% = 97
Sample size (total) = 420

This figure is obtained after taking into consideration of the minimum sample size of 323 and an additional 30% for possibility of non-response rate. A total of 477 samples were recruited in this study.

INCLUSION AND EXCLUSION CRITERIA

Inclusion Criteria

Health professionals (doctors, pharmacists and nurses) who are currently working in the five selected hospitals in Malaysia for at least one year in those hospitals were eligible to be included in this study.

Exclusion Criteria

1. Health professionals who were absent during the data collection process.
2. Health professionals who do not want to be involved in this study.
3. Non-Malaysian citizens.
4. T&CM practitioners.

STUDY INSTRUMENTS

A self-administered questionnaire was used in this study. The study covered two parts namely A and B. Part A was for a quantitative study while part B a qualitative study.

In part A, a self-administered questionnaire was used. In this part, the practice regarding T&CM and related factors were obtained. The questionnaire was in both English and Malay language. In part B, an in-depth semi-structured face-to-face interview was carried out on ten respondents. Two health professionals were selected from each of the hospital. The health professionals included doctors, pharmacists and nurses. The interviews were conducted by the researcher using the English language. This part contained socio-demographic characteristics of the respondents, the practice of T&CM and the idea of integration of T&CM into western medicine (WM). The original questionnaire was in English and it was translated into Malay language as well.

Pre-Test

The questionnaire items were translated into Malay language by a local bilingual translator, who subsequently translated the responses into English language for data processing and analysis.

All study–related information that was relevant to the respondents who have agreed to participate in this study, was distributed to the study participants in the five selected hospitals, endorsed by the National University of Malaysia (UKM), and the Research and Ethics Committee, Faculty of Medicine, UKM. Moreover, the study was also approved by the Malaysian National Institute of Health and the Ministry of Health Malaysia (MOH).

Participants' anonymity and data confidentiality was assured before they participate in the research. The investigator personally explained the main purpose of the study to all including respondents. They were also be informed that all information given in their responses that could identify participants or their households would be treated as confidential, and that the results would be summarized as collective results rather than individual. Moreover, the researcher ensured that all participants fully understood that their given information would be used for research purpose only. Furthermore, the respondents were informed that their participation was voluntary, and that they retained the rights to withdraw their consent at any time should they feel uncomfortable. They were informed that the study posed no risks to them or their families other than that encountered in their everyday life and that they would not be compensated in any way for their participation.

The questionnaire in the Malay language was scrutinized for accuracy and a pilot study performed to guarantee its precision and simplicity before conducting the actual study. A pilot study was conducted on 10% of the sample size (30 respondents) from hospital, to assess research questionnaires, estimate the time needed to perform data collection, in addition to possible difficulties that could be encountered.

Validation Procedures

Two forward translations into Malay language have been done by local bilingual translators who were fluent in both Malay language and English languages. Firstly, English questionnaire was translated into Malay language. This was followed by a reconciliation of the forward translation by other native Malaysian speakers who were not involved in the forward translation process. The basis of the items being translated centered more on the phrase or the actual meaning than on the word-to-word structure thereby ensuring content and conceptual equivalence.

The next step consisted of two back translations of the reconciled Malay language version into English. It was reviewed by five bilingual experts that included linguists and health professionals who selected the most appropriate translation for each item from the reconciled version.

To assure the content validity in terms of coverage and relevance, two independent T&CM experts from a T&CM Division and one T&CM practitioner reviewed the questionnaires and gave useful comments. The questionnaires were also discussed among PhD students, post-doctoral students, and other professors at journal club's meetings. Finally, both the English and the Malay language versions were reviewed again by translators as well as by a health expert.

Reliability

The researcher used an internal consistency check by looking at Cronbach's Alpha Coefficient value which examined the reliability of the questions. For reliability of this study, the overall Cronbach's Alpha was 0.912 with a total number of items equaled to 47. The following table presents the reliability of three domains of T&CM questionnaires.

Cronbach's Alpha reliability coefficient of the following domains is shown in this study for: knowledge about T&CM, attitude towards T&CM, and perception about education in

T&CM were acceptable. The highest Cronbach's Alpha is the attitude at 0.886 from 22 items, followed by perception about education in T&CM at 0.814 from 5 items, and knowledge about T&CM at 0.812 from 20 items respectively.

Table 3.1 Reliability of T&CM Questionnaires

Main Domain	Number of items	Cronbach's alpha
Knowledge about T&CM	20	0.812
Attitude towards T&CM	24	0.886
Perception regarding education in T&CM	5	0.814

SAMPLING FOR QUALITATIVE STUDY

Study Design

A qualitative study was carried out to explore the practice of Traditional and Complementary Medicine among health professionals such as doctors, pharmacists and nurses from five selected hospitals.

Qualitative study was done by way of in-depth semi-structured face-to-face interviews. A total of ten respondents were recruited for this study. The questions and answers during the interview were recorded.

Sampling

Health professionals who has less than one year of working experience, foreigners and who worked at a T&CM unit were excluded from this study. Those who volunteered were given explanation that their voice was going to be recorded and the interview would take approximately 40 - 60 minutes. Each interview was recorded was with respondent's permission. The interview was done using a semi-structured interview format. Almost equal numbers of health professionals were selected from among doctors, pharmacists, and nurses and equal numbers of health professionals selected from each hospital. Overall, three doctors, four pharmacists and three nurses were interviewed from five hospitals, and selection of the same type of health professionals from each hospital was avoided.

From each hospital only two health professionals were interviewed but not two doctors, two pharmacists and two nurses from one hospital. The data obtained were classified into various categories. The interview was done between the period of November 2011 and April 2012.

In-Depth Interview Guide

A semi-structured in-depth interview was used to guide the participants in discussions. The questions asked were as follows:

1. What is your opinion about the use of T&CM in Malaysia? Is it popular among the population?

2. In your opinion, why do people use T&CM? Have you ever used T&CM personally? If yes, what is your reason for using it?
3. Have you ever prescribed or recommended T&CM in the treatment of patients? Why?
4. Do you refer patients to T&CM doctors? Why?
5. Do you believe that T&CM has therapeutic value? Please explain.
6. Do you think that T&CM can be integrated with WM? Please explain.
7. What is your opinion on T&CM being a part of future training for medical students?

Procedures

After the participants were selected according to their eligibility, their participation was confirmed for interview by e-mail or phone call and an appointment for a face-to-face in-depth interview was arranged.

Participants were interviewed for approximately 40-60 minutes at a convenient place at their hospitals. At the beginning of the meeting, the interviewer briefly introduced herself and the purpose of the study, gave some definition about T&CM, reviewed the elements of informed consent and asked the participants to sign the informed consent documents. Participants were given a token of appreciation to compensate for their time. In the middle of the interview, participants took a rest for ten minutes provided with some simple tea break.

The interviewer followed a standardized protocol to ensure that all the interviews were conducted in a similar manner and that an identical set of questions was discussed. The interviewer wrote down notes and audio-taped the conversations. The quality of study also has been approved by the Research and Ethics Committee of Faculty of Medicine, UKM, the Malaysian National Institute of Health and MOH.

Data Analysis

The data obtained were sorted into various categories and analyzed manually due to their small sample size. The themes that were discussed with the participants were namely: main idea about practicing T&CM among general population, using and recommending T&CM, knowledge about T&CM, integrating T&CM into Western Medicine (WM) and opinion about future medical training in T&CM.

Research Ethics

Ethical Committee approvals were obtained from the UKM Medical Center (Ethics Committee/IRB Ref. No: UKM 1.5.3.5/244/SPP3 FF-369-2011), the Malaysian National Institute of Health (Ref No: NMRR-11-857-10102), the Ministry of Health, Malaysia, and all the five selected hospitals respectively.

The privacy of the respondent is very important. Respondents have the rights to know the details of the project, to be explained about why they have been selected, what is the purpose of the study, and that they have the right to refuse, withdraw or avoid answering if they feel uncomfortable. The

respondents of this study read the given documents and gave their consent to participating in the project which should cover all these issues. This research was conducted on a voluntary basis where all respondents were given briefings on the conduct of the study and later they were asked to give their written consent using the Agreement Form.

STUDY VARIABLES

Dependent Variable

The dependent variable is the practice of Traditional and Complementary Medicine (T&CM) among health professionals in five selected hospitals in Malaysia.

Independent Variables

The independent variables are socio-demographic variables such as name of hospital, age, gender, ethnicity, religion, career, years of working, marital status, education level, income, T&CM modalities, knowledge regarding T&CM, attitudes regarding T&CM, reason for practicing T&CM, exposure to T&CM practice, education and training in T&CM, and perception about education in T&CM.

OPERATIONAL DEFINITION OF VARIABLES

Operational Definition of Dependent Variable

Practice of T&CM is defined as either ever used or recommended/prescribed T&CM therapies. It was categorized into use of T&CM during their whole life, in the last one year, referral to the patients or family during their whole life and in the last one year. It was measured by asking whether the health professionals have ever used or recommended/prescribed their family or patients with T&CM in their whole life or in the past one year (respectively) in an internal and external way. It was classified as either user of T&CM or non-user of T&CM.

Operational Definition of Independent Variables

a. Socio-demographic variables

Name of hospital: It is specified as the name of hospital where the respondents are currently working.
Age: Age of respondent at the date of the data collection. It was categorized into four groups (such as 24-29, 30-39, 40-49 and 50 and above).
Gender: Male, female (as recorded by the respondents).
Ethnicity: Malay, Chinese, Indian or other ethnic groups.
Religion: Islam, Buddhism, Christian, Hinduism or others.
Career: It is specified as doctor, nurse or pharmacist.
Years of working: It is defined as years of working in the current hospital at least one year as a health professional. It was further divided into two categories: 10 years and less than 10 years and more than 10 years.
Marital status: Married, single or separated/divorced.
Education level: Diploma, Bachelor, Master and PhD.
Monthly personal income: It was divided into two categories; low income ≤RM 4000, and high income > RM 4000 in a month.

b. Knowledge regarding T&CM

It was measured by using questionnaire on knowledge of T&CM. It covers Malay massage, acupuncture, herbal medicine and Malay postnatal care etc.

Scoring was done by the following steps:

Concerning knowledge, a total of 20 points were scored.

- Scores from 0 to 12 were considered as "poor knowledge"
- Scores from 13 to 20 were be considered as "good knowledge"

c. Attitudes regarding T&CM

Scoring was done in the following steps:

Concerning attitude, a total of 110 points will be scored.

- Scores from 0 to 77 were considered as "negative attitude".
- Scores from 78 to 110 were considered as "positive attitude".

d. Reason for using/recommending T&CM

The reason for using/recommending T&CM is classified into health-related reason and non-health-related reason. Health-related reason is whether the health professionals uses T&CM because of health problem, maintenance of health or both; while non-health related reasons are whether T&CM is considered effective, satisfied, has fewer side effects, cheaper/affordable, philosophically compatible with indigenous culture, familiar with T&CM, failure of western medicine, placebo effect and other reasons.

e. Exposure to T&CM

It is defined as whether health professionals use T&CM because they are influenced by personal experience, family's advice, friend/colleague's advice, mass media or published article, T&CM practitioner's opinion and patient's opinion.

f. Education and training in T&CM

It is defined as whether health professionals attended any workshop, training or conference about T&CM. The answer is categorized into yes or no.

g. T&CM Modalities

It is specified whether health professionals used four main modalities of T&CM such as massage, acupuncture, herbal medicine, postnatal care and other types of T&CM treatments. The answer is categorized into yes or no.

h. Perception about education in T&CM:

Scoring was done in the following steps:

Concerning perception, a total of 5 points were scored.

- Scores from 0 to 3 were considered as "negative perception".
- Scores from 4 to 5 were considered as "positive perception".

DATA COLLECTION AND ANALYSIS

For the purpose of this study, all information was collected by self-administered questionnaire and in-depth interview. Data analysis was carried out using the Statistical Package Of Social Science (SPSS) Version 20. It can be summarized in the following steps:

1. Descriptive statistics, including mean, standard deviation, median, frequency, minimum and maximum were obtained.
2. The prevalence of socio-demographic characteristics of respondents, practice of T&CM, knowledge, attitude towards T&CM, reasons for using T&CM and education in T&CM were compared using the Chi–Squared test (χ^2). The level of significance was taken at $P< 0.05$.
3. The data was normally distributed based on the skewness, kurtosis, histogram and Q-Q pilot results for the Tests of Normality for years of working and personal monthly income respectively.
4. Both bivariate and multivariable analysis (multiple linear regression and logistic regression analysis) were used as a statistical tool in this study.
5. Multiple logistic regression (MLR) analysis was performed in order to obtain estimates adjusted odd

ratios (AORs) of risk factors to practice of T&CM. The practice of T&CM outcome–related variables was selected using a Likelihood Ratio (LR) backward stepwise approach.

6. Bivariate analysis was used to determine the association between the dependent and independent variables. Chi-Square test was used for the qualitative data. The statistical test was considered significant when p-value was less than 0.05. Logistic Regression analysis was used to determine the strength of association between T&CM practice and other associated factors as well as to control the confounders.

Plan for Minimizing Sampling Error and Non-Sampling Error

a. The questionnaire was validated and modified by doing a pilot study.
b. Any question with more than 20% missing data was excluded from the study.
c. Only one researcher recorded the answer from the in-depth interview since the interview for each case took more than 40 minutes. This is to avoid respondent from being tired and to maintain the quality of the answers. Refreshment was provided in between.

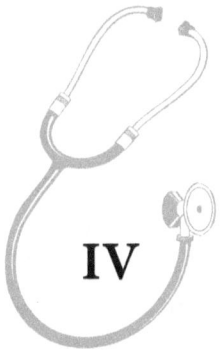

IV

RESULTS

SOCIO-DEMOGRAPHIC FACTORS, KNOWLEDGE, ATTITUDE, PRACTICE OF T&CM, AND REASONS FOR PRACTICING OR NOT PRACTICING T&CM

This study reported the practice of T&CM among health professionals in five selected hospitals in Malaysia. The data were obtained over a period of 10 months from September 2011 to June 2012.

A total of 477 health professionals (respondent rate was 100%) consisting of doctors, pharmacists and nurses were involved in this study. The mean age of participants was 37.4 years old (SD 7.94), minimum age was 24 years old and the maximum age was 56 years old. The minimum and maximum years of working were 2 years and 32 years respectively. Median years of working was 11 years and mean was 13 years. The monthly personal income of participants ranged from RM 2000 to RM 13 000. Median income was RM 5140.

The result of this study reports the practice of T&CM and its associated factors among the health professionals. The study investigated the use of T&CM during whole life, the use of T&CM in the last one year, T&CM referral to patients or family members during a whole life and T&CM referral to patients and family members in the last one year among the health professionals. Modalities of use of T&CM during a whole life, modalities of use of T&CM in the last one year, and T&CM referral to patients or family members during a whole life, as well as T&CM referral in the last one year among health professionals. It also described the level of knowledge and attitude towards T&CM, and perception of education in T&CM. Reasons for practicing or not practicing T&CM were also discussed.

Table 4.1 describes the socio-demographic characteristics of the respondents. The number of respondents from each hospital was almost the same. Majority of them aged between 30 to 49 years old. Male-to-female ratio was 1:3. The majority of the respondents were Malays (58.1%) and Muslims (63.3%). The proportion of doctors and nurses is almost the same but there were fewer pharmacists participated in this study. Majority of the health professionals had more than ten years of working experience. Most of them were married (64.6%) and had a degree (49.5%), and most of the respondents' monthly personal income in this study was less than RM 4,000.

PRACTICE OF TRADITIONAL AND COMPLEMENTARY MEDICINE AMONG HEALTH PROFESSIONALS IN MALAYSIA

Table 4.1 Distribution and socio-demographic characteristics of health professionals (n=477)

Characteristics	No	Percentage (%)
Name of hospitals		
UKMMC	94	19.7
HPJ	90	18.9
HSNZ	96	20.1
HDOK	98	20.5
SGH	99	20.8
Age category (year)		
24-29	83	17.4
30-39	211	44.2
40-49	141	29.6
50 and above	42	8.8
Sex		
Male	108	22.6
Female	369	77.4
Ethnicity		
Malay	277	58.1
Chinese	117	24.5
Indian	11	2.3
Others	72	15.1
Religion		
Islam	302	63.3
Christianity	104	21.8
Buddhism	55	11.5
Hinduism	7	1.5
Others	9	1.9
Career		
Doctors	166	34.8

Pharmacist	142	29.8
Nurse	169	35.4
Years of working		
≤10	215	45.1
>10	262	59.9
Marital Status		
Married	308	64.6
Single	157	32.9
Separated /Divorced/ Widowed	12	2.5
Education level		
Diploma	147	30.8
Degree	236	49.5
Master/PhD	94	19.7
Income category (RM) individual		
Low (≤4000)	253	53.0
High(>4000)	224	47.0

Note: UKMMC=University Kebangsaan Malaysia Medical Center, HPJ=Hospital Putra Jaya, HSNZ=Hospital Sultanah Nur Zahirah, HDOK=Hospital Duchess of Kent, SGH= Sarawak General Hospital.

Table 4.2 Shows that only 13.0% of the respondents have T&CM practitioners in their family.

Table 4.2 Traditional and complementary medicine practitioners in the family

T&CM practitioner	N	Percentage (%)
No	415	87.0
Yes	62	13.0
Total	477	100.0

PRACTICE OF TRADITIONAL AND COMPLEMENTARY MEDICINE AMONG HEALTH PROFESSIONALS IN MALAYSIA

Chart 4.3 shows that a total of 46.3% of the health professionals had ever used T&CM in their lives and 32.5% of them used T&CM in the last one year.

Chart 4.3 Use of T&CM by health professionals

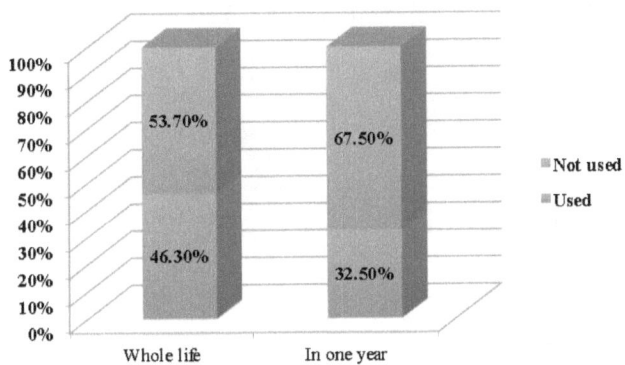

Chart 4.4 shows that 48.6% of the health professionals had ever referred T&CM to their patients or families in their life, and 25.2 % of them referred T&CM in the last one year.

Chart 4.4. Referral of T&CM by health professionals

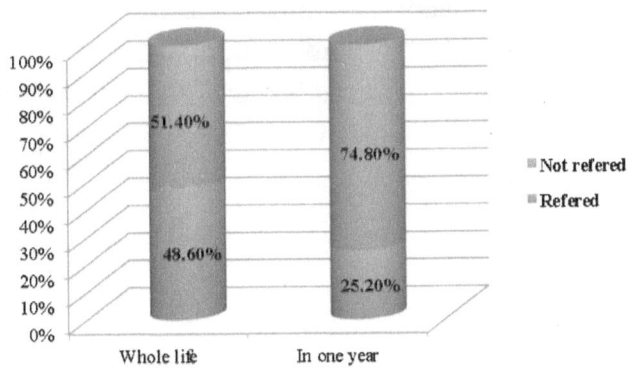

Chart 4.5 shows that a total of 67.5% of the health professionals had ever personally practice (used or recommended) T&CM to their patients and family in their lives and around 46% of them practiced or recommended T&CM to patients and family members in the last one year.

Chart 4.5 Total Use/Referral of T&CM by health professionals

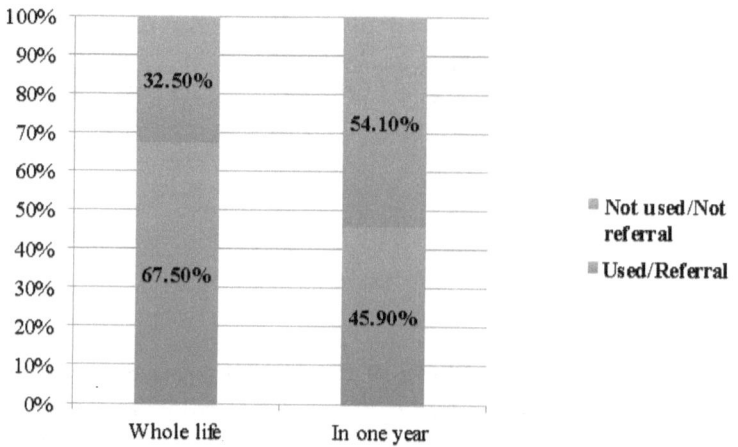

Table 4.6 shows the modalities of T&CM usage wherein almost 20% of respondents have used massage, herbal therapies and postnatal care respectively, while fewer respondents used other types of T&CM (5%) and acupuncture (3.8%) in their lives. However, fewer participants used T&CM in the last one year, in which the use of massage (13.0%) was the highest in comparison to others.

Table 4.6 T&CM modalities used by health professionals

	Yes N (%)	No N (%)	N/A N (%)	Total
Modalities (used whole life)				
Massage	102 (21.4)	375(78.6)		477(100)
Herbal therapies	93 (19.5)	384(80.5)		477(100)
Postnatal care	89 (18.7)	169(35.4)	219(45.9)	477(100)
Others	24 (5.0)	453(95.0)		477(100)
Acupuncture	18 (3.8)	459(96.2)		477(100)
Modalities (in one year)				
Massage	62 (13.0)	415 (87.0)		477 (100)
Herbal therapies	52 (10.9)	425 (89.1)		477 (100)
Postnatal care	39 (8.2)	219 (45.9)	219 (45.9)	477 (100)
Others	17 (3.6)	460 (96.4)		477 (100)
Acupuncture	13 (2.7)	464 (97.3)		477 (100)

Note: N/A=Not applicable (men and unmarried women).

Table 4.7 presents the distribution of respondents according to T&CM referral modalities to the patients and families. More than 30.0% referred to massage and around 13.0% referred to acupuncture and postnatal care in their life respectively. As many as twice the number of respondents (16.4%) referred to massage and acupuncture (8.6%) in the last one year.

Table 4.7 T&CM modalities as referred to by health professionals to patients and families

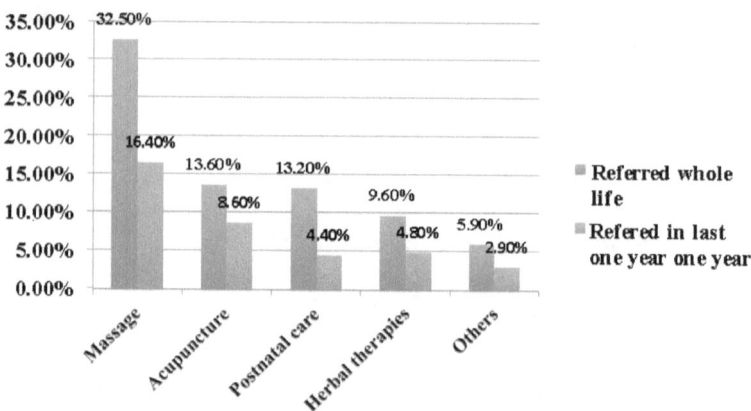

Chart 4.8 shows that 37.7% of the health professionals sometimes asked, 17.2% health professionals rarely asked, 16.6% health professionals never asked, 15.7% health professionals usually asked and only 12.8% health professionals always asked their patients whether they used T&CM or not.

Chart 4.8 Health professionals asked their patients about T&CM usage

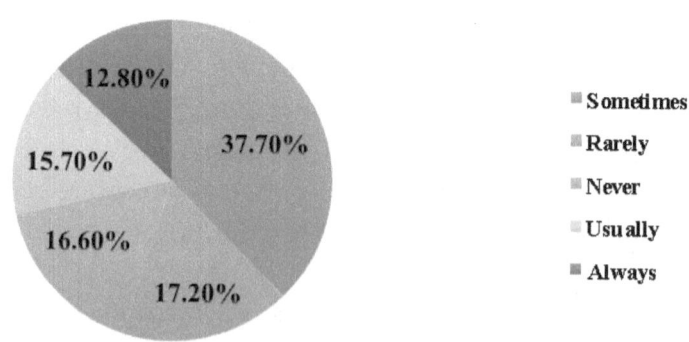

Table 4.9 describes the knowledge of health professionals about T&CM in which a total of 85.1% believed that massage could help in maintaining physical, mental, and emotional well-being, 76.9% believed that T&CM usage was mostly to avoid the side effects of synthetic products, while only 9.0% knew that prickly pear cactus (nopal) was useful for the treatment of diabetes.

Table 4.9 Knowledge about T&CM

Knowledge	Yes N (%)	Unsure N (%)	No N (%)	Total
Due to side effects of synthetic products, natural products are gaining popularity in the market.	367(76.9)	77(16.1)	33(7.0)	477(100.0)
T&CM remedies are useful for chronic illness.	160(33.5)	224 (47.0)	93 (9.5)	477(100.0)
Consumption of Garlic can decrease cholesterol level.	222 (46.5)	211 (44.2)	44 (9.3)	477(100.0)
Consumption of Ginger affects digestive ailments.	250 (52.4)	189 (39.6)	38 (8.0)	477(100.0)

Consumption of Ginkgo helps improve memory and energy.	301 (63.1)	160 (33.5)	16 (3.4)	477(100.0)
Consumption of Ginseng increases energy and virility.	268 (56.2)	191 (40.0)	18 (3.8)	477(100.0)
Consumption of high-dose Ginseng causes hypertension.	138 (28.9)	317 (66.5)	22 (4.6)	477(100.0)
Tongkat Ali is useful for sexual dysfunction.	262 (54.9)	178 (37.3)	37 (7.8)	477(100.0)
Kacip Fatimah is used to maintain a healthy female reproductive system.	313 (65.6)	145 (30.4)	19 (4.0)	477(100.0)
Bitter melon (karela) is useful for the treatment of diabetes mellitus.	190 (39.8)	267 (56.0)	20 (4.2)	477(100.0)
Prickly pear cactus (nopal) is useful for the treatment of diabetes.	43 (9.0)	412 (86.4)	22 (4.6)	477(100.0)

PRACTICE OF TRADITIONAL AND COMPLEMENTARY MEDICINE AMONG HEALTH PROFESSIONALS IN MALAYSIA

Consumption of Green tea can decrease cholesterol level.	236 (49.5)	220 (46.1)	21 (4.4)	477(100.0)
Primrose oil useful for scleroderma.	122 (25.6)	326 (68.3)	29 (6.1)	477(100.0)
Bee pollen enhances the immune system.	252 (52.8)	212 (44.4)	13 (2.8)	477(100.0)
Massage can help you maintain physical and emotional well-being.	406 (85.1)	59 (12.4)	12 (2.5)	477(100.0)
Traditional massage is useful for post-stroke rehabilitation.	347 (72.7)	113 (23.7)	17 (3.6)	477(100.0)
Massage is useful for the treatment of low back pain.	350 (73.4)	102 (21.4)	25(5.2)	477(100.0)
Acupuncture is useful for the treatment of chronic pain.	285 (59.7)	164 (34.4)	28 (5.9)	477(100.0)
Acupuncture is useful for the treatment of stroke.	210 (44.0)	238 (49.9)	29 (6.1)	477(100.0)

Postnatal massage can help to relieve muscle cramps after labour.	364 (76.3)	97 (20.3)	16 (3.4)	477(100.0)

The attitude of the health professionals towards T&CM was collected as is shown in Table 4.10 below. About 73.0% health professionals believed that doctors should have knowledge about T&CM.

Table 4.10 Attitude towards T&CM among the health professionals

	Strongly Disagree N (%)	Disagree N (%)	Unsure N (%)	Agree N (%)	Strongly Agree N (%)	Total N (%)
I believe doctors should have knowledge about T&CM.	2 (0.4)	17 (3.6)	47 (9.9)	347(72.7)	64(13.4)	477(100.0)
Health professionals should advise their patients about using T&CM.	6 (1.3)	58(12.2)	116(24.3)	263(55.1)	34 (7.1)	477(100.0)
T&CM therapies are not a threat to public health.	4 (0.8)	53(11.1)	102(21.4)	26 (56.4)	49(10.3)	477(100.0)
I would use T&CM therapies if they are suitable for me.	5 (1.0)	11 (2.3)	61 (12.8)	326(68.3)	74(15.5)	477(100.0)

PRACTICE OF TRADITIONAL AND COMPLEMENTARY MEDICINE AMONG HEALTH PROFESSIONALS IN MALAYSIA

I would use T&CM if I know about T&CM therapies.	2 (0.4)	13 (2.7)	61 (12.8)	319(66.9)	82(17.2)	477(100.0)
Health professional's knowledge about T&CM practices leads to better patients/clients outcome.	2 (0.4)	8 (1.7)	66 (13.8)	321(67.3)	80(16.8)	477(100.0)
Safe usage of T&CM therapies should be encouraged.	5 (1.0)	23 (4.8)	83 (17.4)	299(62.7)	67(14.0)	477(100.0)
T&CM therapies are generally beneficial for health problem.	2(0.4)	15 (3.1)	158(33.1)	269(56.4)	33 (7.0)	477(100.0)
In some instances of non-threatening disease, I will recommend T&CM.	6 (1.3)	54(11.3)	121(25.4)	272(57.0)	24 (5.0)	477(100.0)
The incorporation of T&CM therapies into the WM.	5 (1.0)	13 (2.7)	169(35.4)	255(53.5)	35 (7.4)	477(100.0)

Health professionals' recommendations of T&CM therapies are influencing the usage of T&CM by the patients.	3 (0.6)	28 (5.9)	123(25.8)	293(61.4)	30 (6.3)	477(100.0)
Mass media should educate the public about T&CM.	3 (0.6)	19(4.0)	73 (15.3)	331(69.4)	51(10.7)	477(100.0)
I would recommend T&CM therapies for some chronic diseases.	5 (1.0)	19 (4.0)	146(30.6)	275(57.7)	32 (6.7)	477(100.0)
I recommend herbal therapies for cancer patients.	28 (5.9)	81 (17)	217(45.5)	135(28.3)	16 (3.3)	477(100.0)
I recommend acupuncture for post-stroke patients.	9 (1.9)	34 (7.1)	206(43.2)	198(41.5)	30 (6.3)	477(100.0)
Traditional postnatal care is beneficial.	6 (1.3)	25 (5.2)	118(24.7)	282(59.1)	46 (9.6)	477(100.0)
I would use T&CM if it is affordable.	6 (1.3)	44 (9.2)	103(21.6)	288(60.4)	36 (7.5)	477(100.0)
I chose T&CM remedy because it is effective.	9 (1.9)	60 (12.6)	202(42.3)	190(39.8)	16 (3.4)	477(100.0)

PRACTICE OF TRADITIONAL AND COMPLEMENTARY MEDICINE AMONG HEALTH PROFESSIONALS IN MALAYSIA

Patients/clients' religious/ spiritual beliefs and practices about T&CM influence me to use T&CM therapies.	15 (3.1)	98 (20.5)	163(34.2)	184(38.6)	17 (3.6)	477(100.0)
I chose T&CM remedy because it has less negative side effects.	14 (2.9)	105(22)	194(40.7)	153(32.)	11 (2.3)	477(100.0)
T&CM therapies stimulate the body's natural therapeutic powers.	6 (1.3)	35 (7.3)	190(39.8)	226(47.4)	20 (4.2)	477 (100)

Chart 4.11 and 4.12 below shows, out of 211 (46.3%) of the health professionals who used T&CM, most of them (50.2%) said they used T&CM to maintain their health, and out of 232 (48.3%) of the health professionals who referred T&CM, most of them (48.3%) said they did so because of both reasons (to maintain health and to treat health problem).

Chart 4.11 Purpose for using T&CM

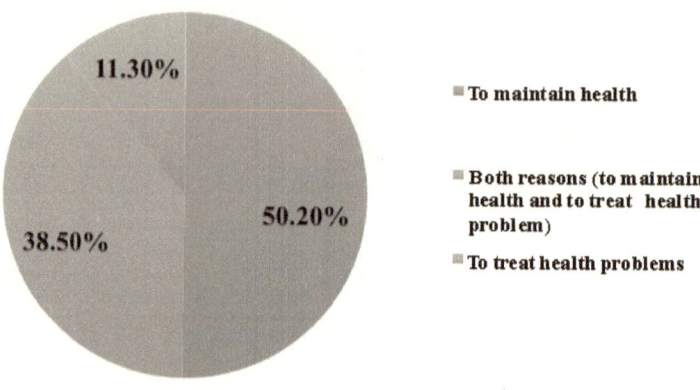

Chart 4.12 Purpose for recommending T&CM

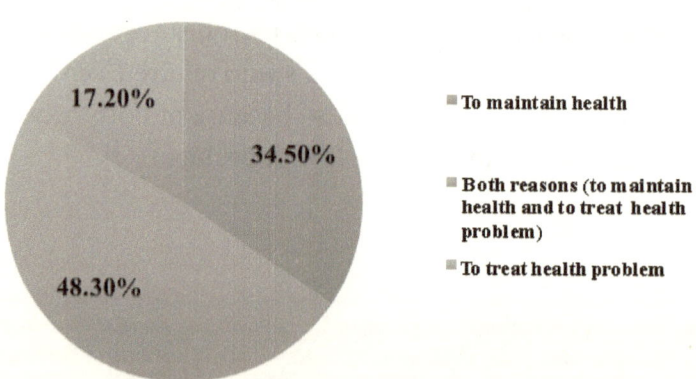

PRACTICE OF TRADITIONAL AND COMPLEMENTARY MEDICINE AMONG HEALTH PROFESSIONALS IN MALAYSIA

Chart 4.13 shows that 44.7% of the health professionals used or recommended T&CM because they believed it was effective, 33.2% said they were satisfied and 28.6% of the respondents believed it had fewer side effects.

Chart 4.13 Reasons for using/recommending T&CM

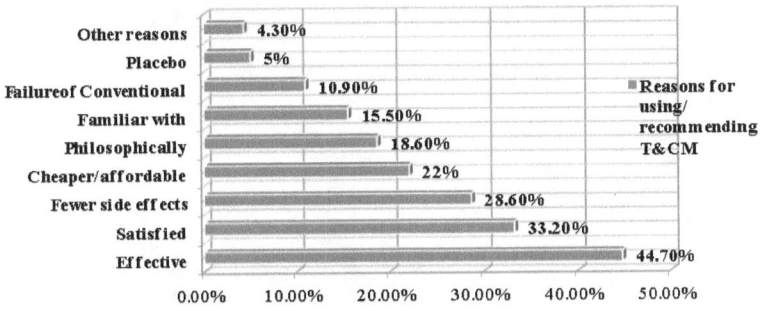

Chart 4.14 shows that most of the health professionals (64.5%) have not used T&CM because they were not familiar with T&CM. Only 3.2% were dissatisfied with T&CM, while 3.9% of them stated that T&CM usage is a failure.

Chart 4.14 Reasons for not using/recommending T&CM

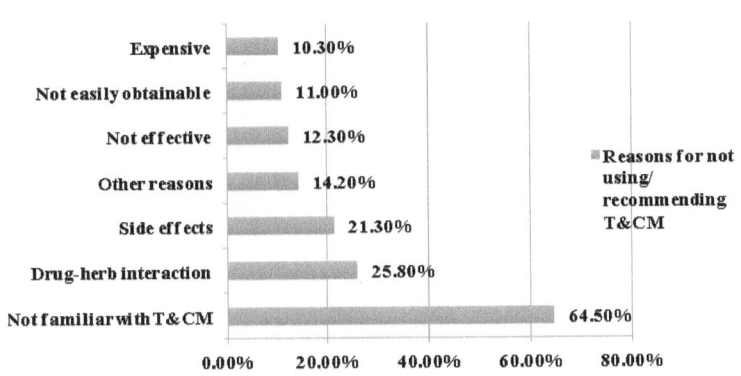

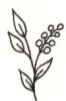

Table 4.15 indicates that most of the health professionals (34.6%) used or recommended T&CM to the patients and families because of their personal experience, followed by family's advice (30.4%), and by friends or colleague's advice (26.2%).

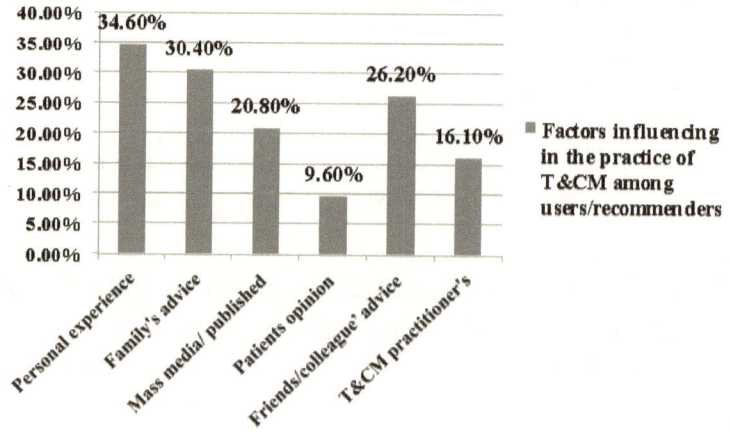

Chart 4.15 Factors influencing in the practice of T&CM among users/recommenders

Table 4.16 describes the education factor in influencing T&CM practices among the health professionals. A total of 21.4% have ever attended some T&CM classes or courses during their study, and 14.5% have joined workshops or conferences in T&CM, and 18.2% mentioned that education and training influenced their practice of T&CM.

Table 4.16 Education in T&CM

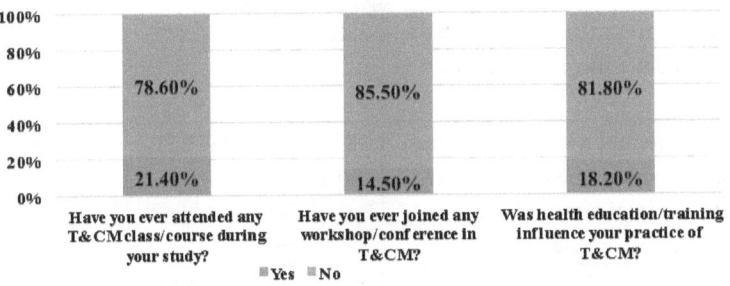

Table 4.17 indicates the perception on education in T&CM. About 89.1 % of the respondents agreed that educational materials about T&CM should be made available at their libraries and bookstores. It is also showed that a total of 83.4% of the respondents agreed that T&CM practitioners have to learn conventional medicine and that the perception about education in T&CM was highly positive among the health professionals.

Table 4.17 Perception on education in T&CM

	Agree N (%)	Unsure N (%)	Disagree N (%)
Educational materials about T&CM should be made available at our libraries and bookstores.	425 (89.1)	41 (8.6)	11 (2.3)
T&CM practitioners have to learn conventional medicine.	398 (83.4)	63 (13.2)	16 (3.4)
Fundamental knowledge about T&CM should be incorporated into medical curriculum.	383 (80.3)	68 (14.2)	26 (5.5)
Education and training in T&CM is important for health professionals.	382 (80.1)	80 (16.8)	15 (3.1)
There should be T&CM advisers or T&CM departments in all hospitals.	376 (78.8)	73 (15.3)	28 (5.9)

Table 4.18 shows the level of knowledge of and attitude towards T&CM and perception on education in T&CM. Knowledge of T&CM among the health professionals was poor (61.2%), however, a majority of them have positive attitude towards T&CM (65.4%) and a positive perception on education in T&CM (85.3%).

Table 4.18 Level of knowledge, attitude towards T&CM and perception on education in T&CM

	N	Percentage (%)
Knowledge regarding T&CM		
Poor	292	61.2
Good	185	38.8
Attitude regarding T&CM		
Positive	312	65.4
Negative	165	34.6
Perception about education in T&CM		
Positive	407	85.3
Negative	70	14.7
Total	477	100.0

RELATIONSHIP BETWEEN SOCIO-DEMOGRAPHIC CHARACTERISTICS OF HEALTH PROFESSIONALS AND THEIR USE OF T&CM AND T&CM REFERRAL TO PATIENTS AND FAMILY

In this part of the analysis, a chi-squared test explores the relationship between the practice of T&CM and its associated factors. Table 4.19 shows the association between the use of T&CM during whole life and socio-demographic characteristics of the respondents. This finding shows that female (49.9%) used significantly higher T&CM in their whole life as compared to male health professionals (34.3%) (p=0.004). Nurses (56.2%), health professionals who have more than 10 years of working experience (50.8%), and married health professionals (52.3%) used significantly higher T&CM in their lives as compared to pharmacists, doctors with working experience less than 10 years, and health professionals who are not married (p=0.005, p=0.032, and p<0.001 respectively).

There was no significant difference in the use of T&CM in whole life between hospitals, age group, ethnicity, religion, education level and income among the health professionals.

Table 4.19 Socio-demographic characteristics and use of T&CM during the whole life among the health professionals.

T&CM Used (Whole life)	Used N (%) 221(46.3)	Not Used N(%) 256(53.7)	Total =477	X^2	p-value
Hospitals				4.73	0.316
UKMMC	37 (39.4)	57 (60.6)	94		
HPJ	37 (41.1)	53 (58.9)	90		
HSNZ	49 (51.0)	47 (49.0)	96		
HDOK	50 (51.0)	48 (49.0)	98		
SGH	48 (48.5)	51 (51.5)	99		
Age (year)				1.377	0.241
<40	130 (44.2)	164 (55.8)	294		
≥40	91 (49.7)	92 (50.3)	183		
Sex				8.182	0.004**
Male	37 (34.3)	71 (65.7)	108		
Female	184(49.9)	185 (50.1)	369		

Ethnicity				0.245	0.620
Malay	131 (47.3)	146 (52.7)	277		
Non-Malay	90 (45.0)	110 (55.0)	200		
Religion				0.604	0.437
Islam	144 (47.7)	158 (52.3)	302		
Non- Islam	77 (44.0)	98 (56.0)	175		
Career				10.723	0.005**
Doctors	65 (39.2)	101 (60.8)	166		
Pharmacists	61 (43.0)	81 (57.0)	142		
Nurses	95 (56.2)	74 (43.8)	169		
Years of working				4.592	0.032*
≤10	88 (40.9)	127 (59.1)	215		
>10	133(50.8)	129 (49.2)	262		
Marital Status				12.342	<0.001***
Married	161(52.3)	147 (47.7)	308		
Not married	60 (35.5)	109 (64.5)	169		
Education Level				0.469	0.791
Diploma	69 (46.9)	78 (53.1)	147		
Degree	106(44.9)	130 (55.1)	236		
Master/PhD	46 (48.9)	48 (51.1)	94		
Income(RM)				3.239	0.072
Low(<4000)	127(50.2)	126 (49.8)	253		
High(≥4000)	94 (42.0)	130 (58.0)	224		

*Significant at p<0.05, **Significant at p<0.01, ***Significant at p<0.001

Table 4.20 shows the association between the practice of T&CM and socio-demographic characteristics of the respondents in west and east Malaysia. There is no significant difference between hospitals in west and east Malaysia and use of T&CM in whole life, in the last one year, referral of T&CM in whole life and in the last one year.

Table 4.20 Association between the practice of T&CM and health professionals in west and east Malaysia

	Yes N(%)	No N(%)	Total	X^2	p-value
T&CM Used (in whole Life)					
Hospitals	221 (46.3)	256(53.7)	477	1.574	0.210
in West Malaysia	123 (43.9)	157(56.1)	280		
in East Malaysia	98 (49.7)	99 (50.3)	197		
T&CM Used (in the last one year)					
Hospitals	155 (32.5)	322(67.5)	477	0.000	0.998
In West Malaysia	91 (32.5)	189(67.5)	280		
In East Malaysia	64 (32.5)	133(67.5)	197		
T&CM Referral (in whole Life)					
Hospitals	232 (48.6)	245 (51.4)	477	0.274	0.600
in West Malaysia	139 (49.6)	141 (50.4)	280		
in East Malaysia	93 (47.2)	104 (52.8)	197		

T&CM Referral (in the last one year)					
Hospitals	120 (25.2)	357 (74.8)	477	1.905	0.168
in West Malaysia	64 (22.9)	216 (77.1)	280		
in East Malaysia	56 (28.4)	141 (71.6)	197		

Table 4.21 shows the association between the practice of T&CM and socio-demographic characteristics of the respondents. There is no significant difference between specialist and non-specialist doctors and use/referral of T&CM, use of T&CM in whole life, in the last one year, referral T&CM in whole life and in the last one year.

Table 4.21 Association between the use/referral of T&CM and specialist and non-specialist doctors

	Yes N (%)	No N (%)	Total	X^2	p-value
T&CM used/ referral (in whole life)					
Doctors	108 (65.1)	58 (34.9)	166	0.732	0.392
Non-specialist	88 (66.7)	44 (33.3)	132		
Specialist	20 (58.8)	14 (41.2)	34		

T&CM used (in whole life)					
Doctors	65 (39.2)	101 (60.8)	166	1.704	0.192
Non-specialist	55 (41.7)	77 (58.3)	132		
Specialist	10 (29.4)	24 (70.6)	34		
T&CM used (in the last one year)					
Doctors	52 (31.3)	114 (68.7)	166	2.291	0.130
Non-specialist	45 (34.1)	87 (65.9)	132		
Specialist	7 (20.6)	27 (79.4)	34		
T&CM referral (in whole life)					
Doctors	78 (47.0)	88 (53.0)	166	0.141	0.707
Non-specialist	63 (47.7)	69 (52.3)	132		
Specialist	15 (44.1)	19 (55.9)	34		
T&CM referral (in the last one year)					
Doctors	119 (28.3)	47 (71.7)	166	0.072	0.789
Non-specialist	38 (28.8)	94 (71.2)	132		
Specialist	9 (26.5)	25 (73.5)	34		

Table 4.22 shows the association between the use of T&CM in the last one year and socio-demographic characteristics of the respondents. The finding shows that females (36.0%) (p=0.002), Malays (36.1%), Muslims (36.1%) and married health professionals (36.0%) were more likely to use T&CM as compared to males, non-Malays, non-Muslims and non married health professionals in the last one year (p=0.0048, p=0.028 and p=0.026 respectively). There was no significant difference between hospitals, age, career, working experience, education level, income and use of T&CM in the last one year.

Table 4.22 Socio-demographic characteristics and use of T&CM in the last year among the health professionals

T&CM Used (One year)	Used N (%) 155(32.5)	Not Used N (%) 322 (67.5)	Total=477	X^2	p-value
Hospitals				1.019	0.907
UKMMC	29 (30.9)	65 (69.1)	94		
HPJ	29 (32.2)	61 (67.8)	90		
HSNZ	33 (34.4)	63 (65.6)	96		
HDOK	29 (29.6)	69 (70.4)	98		
SGH	35 (35.4)	64 (64.6)	99		
Age (year)				0.095	0.758
<40	94 (32.0)	200 (68.0)	294		
≥40	61 (33.3)	122 (66.7)	183		
Sex				9.356	0.002**
Male	22 (20.4)	86 (79.6)	108		
Female	133 (36.0)	236 (64.0)	369		
Ethnicity				3.917	0.048*
Malay	100 (36.1)	177 (63.9)	277		

Non Malay	55 (27.5)	145 (72.5)	200		
Religion				4.858	0.028*
Islam	109 (36.1)	193 (63.9)	302		
Non-Islam	46 (26.3)	129 (73.7)	175		
Career				1.118	0.572
Doctors	52 (31.3)	114 (68.7)	166		
Pharmacists	43 (30.3)	99 (69.7)	142		
Nurses	60 (35.5)	109 (64.5)	169		
Years of working				0.913	0.339
≤10	65 (30.2)	150 (69.8)	215		
>10	90 (34.4)	172 (65.6)	262		
Marital Status				4.978	0.026*
Married	111 (36.0)	197 (64.0)	308		
Not married	44 (26.0)	125 (74.0)	169		
Education Level				0.03	0.985
Diploma	47 (32.0)	100 (68.0)	147		
Degree	77 (32.6)	159 (67.4)	236		
Master/PhD	31 (33.0)	63 (67.0)	94		
Income(RM)				0.024	0.877
Low(<4000)	83 (32.8)	170 (67.2)	253		
High(≥4000)	72 (32.1)	152 (67.9)	224		

*Significant at $p<0.05$, **Significant at $p<0.01$

Table 4.23 shows the association between T&CM referral during whole life and socio-demographic characteristics of the respondents. The finding shows that the health professionals aged 40 years and older (55.7%), Muslims (53.0%) and health professionals who have more than 10 years of working experience (55.3%) were more likely to refer patients or their family members to T&CM ($p=0.014$, $p=0.013$

and p=0.001 respectively). There was no significant difference T&CM referral in their lives between hospitals, sex, ethnicity, career, working experience, marital status, education, level and income.

Table 4.23 Socio-demographic characteristics and referral T&CM during whole life among the health professionals

T&CM Referral (Whole Life)	Referred N(%) 232(48.6)	Not Referred N (%) 245 (51.4)	Total=477	X²	p- Value
Hospitals				8.366	0.079
UKMMC	37 (39.4)	57 (60.6)	94		
HPJ	54 (60.0)	36 (40.0)	90		
HSNZ	48 (50.0)	48 (50.0)	96		
HDOK	48 (49.0)	50 (51.0)	98		
SGH	45 (45.5)	54 (54.5)	99		
Age (year)				5.992	0.014*
<40	130(44.2)	164 (55.8)	294		
≥40	102(55.7)	81 (44.3)	183		
Sex				0.011	0.918
Male	53 (49.1)	55 (50.9)	108		
Female	179(48.5)	190 (51.5)	369		
Ethnicity				3.639	0.056
Malay	145(52.3)	132(47.7)	277		
Non-Malay	87(43.5)	113(56.5)	200		
Religion				6.215	0.013*
Islam	160(53.0)	142(47.0)	302		
Non-Islam	72(41.1)	103(58.9)	175		
Career				3.864	0.145

Doctors	78(47.0)	88(53.0)	166		
Pharmacists	62(43.7)	80(56.3)	142		
Nurses	92(54.4)	77(45.6)	169		
Years of working				10.464	0.001**
≤10	87(40.5)	128(59.5)	215		
>10	145(55.3)	117(44.7)	262		
Marital Status				4.469	0.107
Married	157 (51.0)	151 (49.0)	308		
Not married	75 (44.4))	94 (55.6)	169		
Education Level				2.833	0.243
Diploma	68(46.3)	79 (53.7)	147		
Degree	111 (47.0)	125 (53.0)	236		
Master/PhD	53 (56.4)	41 (43.6)	94		
Income (RM)				0.314	0.575
Low (<4000)	120 (47.4)	133 (52.6)	253		
High (≥4000)	112 (50.0)	112 (50.0)	224		

*Significant at $p<0.05$, **Significant at $p<0.01$

Table 4.24 shows the association between T&CM referral in the last one year and socio demographic characteristics of the respondents.

The finding shows that male health professionals (36.1%) were more likely to refer patients or their family members to T&CM ($p=0.003$) as compared to female health professionals. There was no significant difference in T&CM referral between hospitals, age, ethnicity, religion, career, working experience, marital status, education level, income and T&CM referral in the last one year.

Table 4.24 Socio-demographic characteristics and referral T&CM in the last one yea among the health professionals

T&CM Referral (One Year)	Referred =232(48.6) N (%)	Not Referred =245 (51.4) N (%)	Total =477	X^2	p-value
Hospitals				4.965	0.291
UKMMC	16 (17.0)	78 (83.0)	94		
HPJ	25 (27.8)	65 (72.2)	90		
HSNZ	23 (24.0)	73 (76.0)	96		
HDOK	29 (29.6)	69 (70.4)	98		
SGH	27 (27.3)	72 (72.7)	99		
Age (year)				2.985	0.084
<40	66 (22.4)	228 (77.6)	294		
≥40	54 (29.5)	129 (70.5)	183		
Sex				8.897	0.003**
Male	39 (36.1)	69 (63.9)	108		
Female	81 (22.0)	288 (78.0)	369		
Ethnicity				0.502	0.478
Malay	73 (26.4)	204 (73.6)	277		
Non-Malay	47 (23.5)	153 (76.5)	200		
Religion				0.439	0.508
Islam	79 (26.2)	223 (73.8)	302		
Non- Islam	41 (23.4)	134 (76.6)	175		
Career				1.469	0.480
Doctors	47 (28.3)	119 (71.7)	166		
Pharmacists	32 (22.5)	110 (77.5)	142		
Nurses	41 (24.3)	128 (75.7)	169		
Years of working				2.26	0.133

≤10	47 (21.9)	168 (78.1)	215		
>10	73 (27.9)	189 (72.1)	262		
Marital Status				0.011	0.915
Married	77 (25.0)	231 (75.0)	308		
Not married	43 (25.4)	126 (74.6)	169		
Education Level				0.945	0.623
Diploma	33 (22.4)	114 (77.6)	147		
Degree	61 (25.8)	175 (74.2)	236		
Master/PhD	26 (27.7)	68 (72.3)	94		
Income (RM)				3.343	0.067
Low (<4000)	55 (21.7)	198 (78.3)	253		
High (≥4000)	65 (29.0)	159 (71.0)	224		

** Significant at p<0.01

Table 4.25 shows the association between the use of massage during whole life and socio-demographic characteristics of the respondents. The finding shows that at the five selected hospitals, the use of massage was significantly higher among the health professionals in Hospital Duchess of Kent (31.6%) (p=0.045) among nurses (29%) and married health professionals (25.6%) (p=0.009 and p=0.002 respectively). There was no significant difference in use of massage in the whole life between age, sex, ethnicity, religion, working experience, education level and income among the health professionals.

Table 4.25 Socio-demographic characteristics and use of massage during a whole life among the health professionals

PRACTICE OF TRADITIONAL AND COMPLEMENTARY MEDICINE AMONG HEALTH PROFESSIONALS IN MALAYSIA

Massage	Used =102(21.4) N (%)	Not Used =375(78.6) N (%)	Total=477	X^2	p-value
Hospitals				9.741	0.045*
UKMMC	21 (22.3)	73 (77.7)	94		
HPJ	17 (18.9)	73 (81.1)	90		
HSNZ	19 (19.8)	77 (80.2)	96		
HDOK	31 (31.6)	67 (68.4)	98		
SGH	14 (14.1)	85 (85.9)	99		
Age (year)				1.816	0.178
<40	57 (19.4)	237 (80.6)	294		
≥40	45 (24.6)	138 (75.4)	183		
Sex				0.312	0.576
Male	21 (19.4)	87 (80.6)	108		
Female	81 (22.0)	288 (78.0)	369		
Ethnicity				1.164	0.281
Malay	64 (23.1)	213 (76.9)	277		
Non-Malay	38 (19.0)	162 (81.0)	200		
Religion				2.214	0.137
Islam	71 (23.5)	231 (76.5)	302		
Non-Islam	31 (17.7)	144 (82.3)	175		
Career				9.529	0.009**
Doctors	26 (15.7)	140 (84.3)	166		
Pharmacists	27 (19.0)	115 (81.0)	142		
Nurses	49 (29.0)	120 (71.0)	169		
Years of working				3.204	0.073
≤10	38 (17.7)	177 (82.3)	215		
>10	64 (24.4)	198 (75.6)	262		
Marital Status				9.41	0.002**
Married	79 (25.6)	229 (74.4)	308		

Not married	23 (13.6)	146 (86.4)	169		
Education Level				1.836	0.399
Diploma	37 (25.2)	110 (74.8)	147		
Degree	47 (19.9)	189 (80.1)	236		
Master/PhD	18 (19.1)	76 (80.9)	94		
Income (RM)				0.761	0.383
Low (<4000)	58 (22.9)	195 (77.1)	253		
High (≥4000)	44 (19.6)	180 (80.4)	224		

*Significant at p<0.05, **Significant at p<0.01

Table 4.26 shows the association between use of acupuncture during a whole life and socio-demographic characteristics of the respondent. The respondents' use of acupuncture was significantly higher among the non-Malays (7.4%) (p=0.002 and p=0.001 respectively). There was no significant difference in use of acupuncture during whole life among health professionals between hospitals, age, sex, career, working experience, marital status, education level and income.

Table 4.26 Socio-demographic characteristics and use of acupuncture during a whole life among the health professionals

Acupuncture	Used =18(3.8%) N (%)	Not Used =459(96.2%) N (%)	Total =477	X^2	p-value
Hospitals				3.342	0.502
UKMMC	3 (3.2)	91 (96.8)	94		
HPJ	2 (2.2)	88 (97.8)	90		
HSNZ	2 (2.1)	94 (94.9)	96		

PRACTICE OF TRADITIONAL AND COMPLEMENTARY MEDICINE AMONG HEALTH PROFESSIONALS IN MALAYSIA

HDOK	5 (5.1)	93 (94.9)	98		
SGH	6 (6.1)	93 (93.9)	99		
Age (year)				0.002	0.963
<40	11 (3.7)	283 (96.3)	294		
≥40	7 (3.8)	176 (96.2)	183		
Sex				0.002	0.965
Male	4 (3.7)	104 (96.3)	108		
Female	14 (3.8)	355 (96.2)	369		
Ethnicity				9.873	0.002**
Malays	4 (1.4)	273 (98.6)	277		
Non-Malays	14 (7.0)	186 (93.0)	200		
Religion				10.169	0.001**
Islam	5 (1.7)	297 (98.3)	302		
Non-Islam	13 (7.4)	162 (92.6)	175		
Career				0.811	0.667
Doctors	5 (3.0)	161 (97.0)	166		
Pharmacists	7 (4.9)	135 (95.1)	142		
Nurses	6 (3.6)	163 (96.4)	169		
Years of working				1.041	0.307
≤10	6 (2.8)	209 (97.2)	215		
>10	12 (4.6)	250 (95.4)	262		
Marital Status				1.736	0.188
Married	9 (2.9)	299 (97.1)	308		
Not married	9 (5.3)	160 (94.7)	169		
Education Level				0.127	0.938
Diploma	6 (4.1)	141 (95.9)	147		
Degree	9 (3.8)	227 (96.2)	236		
Master/PhD	3 (3.2)	91 (96.8)	94		
Income (RM)				0.489	0.484

Low (<4000)	11 (4.3)	242 (95.7)	253		
High (≥4000)	7 (3.1)	217 (96.9)	224		

** Significant at p<0.01

Table 4.27 shows the association between the use of herbal medicine during whole life and socio-demographic characteristics of the respondents. The finding shows that there was no significant difference in the use of herbal medicine during whole life among the health professionals between hospitals, age, sex, ethnicity, religion, career, working experience, marital status, education level and income.

Table 4.27 Socio-demographic characteristics and use of herbal medicine during a whole life among the health professionals

Herbal Medicine	Used =93(19.5%) N (%)	Not Used =384(80.5) N (%)	Total=477	X^2	p-value
Hospitals				0.843	0.933
UKMMC	17 (18.1)	77 (81.9)	94		
HPJ	16 (17.8)	74 (82.2)	90		
HSNZ	18 (18.8)	78 (81.2)	96		
HDOK	20 (20.4)	78 (79.6)	98		
SGH	22 (22.2)	77 (77.8)	99		
Age (year)				0.304	0.581
<40	55 (18.7)	239 (81.3)	294		
≥40	38 (20.8)	145 (79.2)	183		
Sex				2.797	0.094
Male	15 (13.9)	93 (86.1)	108		
Female	78 (21.1)	291 (78.9)	369		

Ethnicity				0.496	0.481
Malays	51 (18.4)	226 (81.6)	277		
Non- Malays	42 (21.0)	158 (79.0)	200		
Religion				0.045	0.833
Islam	58 (19.2)	244 (80.8)	302		
Non-Islam	35 (20.0)	140 (80.0)	175		
Career				2.864	0.239
Doctors	26 (15.7)	140 (84.3)	166		
Pharmacists	33 (23.2)	109 (76.8)	142		
Nurses	34 (20.1)	135 (79.9)	169		
Years of working				0.045	0.831
≤10	41 (19.1)	174 (80.9)	215		
>10	52 (19.8)	210 (80.2)	262		
Marital Status				0.064	0.800
Married	59 (19.2)	249 (80.8)	308		
Not married	34 (20.1)	135 (79.9)	169		
Education Level				1.354	0.508
Diploma	29 (19.7)	118 (80.3)	147		
Degree	42 (17.8)	194 (82.2)	236		
Master/PhD	22 (23.4)	72 (76.6)	94		
Income (RM)				2.388	0.122
Low (<4000)	56 (22.1)	197 (77.9)	253		
High (≥4000)	37 (16.5)	187 (83.5)	224		

Table 4.28 shows the association between the use of postnatal care during whole life and socio-demographic characteristics of the respondents. The finding shows that the use of postnatal care was significantly higher in Hospital Putrajaya (46.3%) and among Malay health professionals (38.9%) (p=0.03 and

p=0.032 respectively). There was no significant difference in the use of postnatal care during whole life among the health professionals between age, religion, career, working experience, marital status, education level and income.

Table 4.28 Socio-demographic characteristics and use of postnatal care during a whole life among married female health professionals

Postnatal Care (Married female)	Used =89(34.5%) N (%)	Not Used =169(65.5%) N (%)	Total=258	X^2	p-value
Hospitals				10.715	0.030*
UKMMC	10 (18.9)	43 (81.1)	53		
HPJ	25 (46.3)	29 (53.7)	54		
HSNZ	27 (40.3)	40 (59.7)	67		
HDOK	14 (35.9)	25 (64.1)	39		
SGH	13 (28.9)	32 (71.1)	45		
Age (year)				1.691	0.193
<40	43 (30.9)	96 (69.1)	139		
≥40	46 (38.7)	73 (61.3)	119		
Ethnicity				4.578	0.032*
Malays	68 (38.9)	107 (61.1)	175		
Non Malays	21 (25.3)	62 (74.7)	169		
Religion				3.279	0.070
Islam	71 (37.8)	117 (62.2)	188		
Non Islam	18 (25.7)	52 (25.7)	70		
Career				1.878	0.391
Doctors	29 (40.3)	43 (59.7)	72		
Pharmacists	14 (28.6)	35 (71.5)	49		
Nurses	46 (33.6)	91 (66.4)	137		

				0.305	0.581
Years of working					
≤10	27 (32.1)	57 (67.9)	84		
>10	62 (35.6)	112 (64.4)	174		
Marital Status				1.768	0.184
Married	88 (35.2)	162 (64.8)	250		
Not married	1 (12.5)	7 (87.5)	8		
Education Level				3.689	0.158
Diploma	28 (33.7)	55 (66.3)	83		
Degree	37 (30.3)	85 (69.7)	122		
Master/PhD	24 (45.3)	29 (54.7)	53		
Income (RM)				0.154	0.694
Low (<4000)	46 (35.7)	83 (64.3)	129		
High (≥4000)	43 (33.3)	86 (66.7)	129		

*Significant at p<0.05

Table 4.29 shows the association between the use of other types of T&CM during whole life and socio-demographic characteristics of the respondents. The finding shows that male health professionals (9.3%) were more likely to use other types of T&CM in their whole life (p=0.022) as compared to female health professionals. There was no significant difference between hospitals, age, ethnicity, religion, career, working experience, marital status, education level, income and the use of other types of T&CM during whole life among the health professionals.

Table 4.29 Socio-demographic characteristics and use of other types of T&CM during a whole life among the health professionals

 DR. MAGFIRET A. BOZLAR, PROF. DR. SYED ALJUNID

Other Types of T&CM	Used =24(5.0%) N (%)	Not Used =453(95.0%) N (%)	Total =477	X^2	p-value
Hospitals				5.453	0.244
UKMMC	4 (4.3)	90 (95.7)	94		
HPJ	2 (2.2)	88 (97.8)	90		
HSNZ	8 (8.3)	88 (91.7)	96		
HDOK	3 (3.1)	95 (96.9)	98		
SGH	7 (7.1)	92 (92.9)	99		
Age (year)				3.285	0.070
<40	19 (6.5)	275 (93.5)	294		
≥40	5 (2.7)	178 (97.3)	183		
Sex				5.222	0.022*
Male	10 (9.3)	98 (90.7)	108		
Female	14 (3.8)	355 (96.2)	369		
Ethnicity				0.767	0.381
Malay	16 (5.8)	261 (94.2)	277		
Non-Malay	8 (4.0)	192 (96.0)	200		
Religion				0.615	0.433
Islam	17 (5.6)	285 (94.4)	302		
Non Islam	7 (4.0)	168 (96.0)	175		
Career				4.297	0.117
Doctors	12 (7.2)	154 (92.8)	166		
Pharmacists	8 (5.6)	134 (94.4)	142		
Nurses	4 (2.4)	165 (97.6)	169		
Years of working				0.248	0.619
≤10	12 (5.6)	203 (94.4)	215		
>10	12 (4.6)	250 (95.4)	262		
Marital Status				2.345	0.126

Married	12 (3.9)	296 (96.1)	308		
Non married	12 (7.1)	157 (92.9)	169		
Education Level				0.797	0.671
Diploma	6 (4.1)	141 (95.9)	147		
Degree	14 (5.9)	222 (94.1)	236		
Master/PhD	4 (4.3)	90 (95.7)	94		
Income (RM)				0.013	0.91
Low (<4000)	13 (5.1)	240 (94.9)	253		
High (≥4000)	11 (4.9)	213 (95.1)	224		

*Significant at p<0.05

Table 4.30 shows the association between the use of massage in the last one year and socio-demographic characteristic of the respondents. The finding shows that nurses (32.0%) and married health professionals (15.6%) were more likely to use massage in the last one year (p=0.011 and p=0.023 respectively). There was no significant difference in the use of massage in the last one year among health professionals between hospitals, age, sex, ethnicity, religion, working experience, education level and income.

Table 4.30 Socio-demographic characteristics and use of massage in the last one year among the health professionals

Massage (in the last one year)	Used =62(13.0%) N (%)	Not Used =415(87.0%) N (%)	Total =477	X²	p-value
Hospitals				2.032	0.730
UKMMC	13 (13.8)	81 (86.2)	94		
HPJ	9 (10.0)	81 (90.0)	90		

HSNZ	16 (16.7)	80 (83.3)	96		
HDOK	12 (12.2)	86 (87.8)	98		
SGH	12 (12.1)	87 (87.9)	99		
Age (year)				3.027	0.082
<40	32 (10.9)	262 (89.1)	294		
≥40	30 (16.4)	153 (83.6)	183		
Sex				2.686	0.101
Male	9 (8.3)	99 (91.7)	108		
Female	53 (14.4)	316 (85.6)	369		
Ethnicity				2.737	0.098
Malay	42 (15.2)	235 (84.8)	277		
Non-Malay	20 (10.0)	180 (90.0)	200		
Religion				3.633	0.057
Islam	46 (15.2)	256 (84.8)	302		
Non Islam	16 (9.1)	159 (90.9)	175		
Career				9.084	0.011*
Doctors	19 (11.4)	147 (88.6)	166		
Pharmacists	11 (7.7)	131 (92.3)	142		
Nurses	32 (18.9)	137 (81.1)	169		
Years of working				2.647	0.104
≤10	22 (10.2)	193 (89.8)	215		
>10	40 (15.3)	222 (84.7)	262		
Marital Status				5.143	0.023*
Married	48 (15.6)	260 (84.4)	308		
Not married	14 (8.3)	155 (91.7)	169		
Education Level				0.776	0.678
Diploma	22 (15.0)	125 (85.0)	147		
Degree	28 (11.9)	208 (88.1)	236		
Master/PhD	12 (12.8)	82 (87.2)	94		

Income (RM)				0.619	0.431
Low (<4000)	30 (11.9)	223 (88.1)	253		
High (≥4000)	32 (14.3)	192 (85.7)	224		

*significant at p<0.05

Table 4.31 shows the association between the use of acupuncture in the last one year and socio-demographic characteristics of the respondents. The finding shows that non-Malays (5.0%), non-Muslims (5.7%) and married health professionals (5.3%) were more likely to use acupuncture in the last one year (p=0.01, p=0.002 and P=0.01 respectively). There was no significant difference in the use of acupuncture in the last one year among health professionals between hospitals, age, sex, career, working experience, education level and income.

Table 4.31 Socio-demographic characteristics and use of acupuncture in the last one year among the health professionals

Acupuncture (in the last one year)	Used =13(2.7%) N (%)	Not Used =464(97.3%) N (%)	Total =477	X^2	p-value
Hospitals				7.724	0.102
UKMMC	1 (1.1)	93 (98.9)	94		
HPJ	1 (1.1)	89 (98.9)	90		
HSNZ	1 (1.0)	95 (99.0)	96		
HDOK	4 (4.1)	94 (95.9)	98		
SGH	6 (6.1)	93 (93.9)	99		
Age (year)				0.343	0.558
<40	7 (2.4)	287 (97.6)	294		

≥40	6 (3.3)	177 (96.7)	183		
Sex				0.504	0.478
Male	4 (3.7)	104 (96.3)	108		
Female	9 (2.4)	360 (97.6)	369		
Ethnicity				6.722	0.010*
Malays	3 (1.1)	274 (98.9)	277		
Non-Malays	10 (5.0)	190 (95.0)	200		
Religion				9.314	0.002**
Islam	3 (1.0)	299 (99.0)	302		
Non-Islam	10 (5.7)	165 (94.3)	175		
Career				0.138	0.933
Doctors	5 (3.0)	161 (97.0)	166		
Pharmacists	4 (2.8)	138 (97.2)	142		
Nurses	4 (2.4)	165 (97.6)	169		
Years of working				0.236	0.627
≤10	5 (2.3)	210 (97.7)	215		
>10	8 (3.1)	254 (96.9)	262		
Marital Status				6.674	0.010*
Married	4 (1.3)	304 (98.7)	308		
Not married	9 (5.3)	160 (94.7)	169		
Education Level				0.780	0.677
Diploma	3 (2.0)	144 (98.0)	147		
Degree	8 (3.4)	228 (96.6)	236		
Master/PhD	2 (2.1)	92 (97.9)	94		
Income (RM)				3.061	0.080
Low (<4000)	10 (4.0)	243 (96.0)	253		
High (≥4000)	3 (1.3)	221 (98.7)	224		

*significant at p<0.05, **significant at p<0.01

Table 4.32 shows the association between the use of herbal medicine in the last one year and socio-demographic characteristics of the respondents. The finding shows that there was no significant difference in the use of herbal medicine in the last one year among health professionals between hospitals, age, sex, ethnicity, religion, career, working experience, education level and income.

Table 4.32 Socio-demographic characteristics and use of herbal medicine in the last one year among the health professionals

Herbal Medicine (in the last one year)	Used =52(10.9%) N (%)	Not Used =425(89.1%) N (%)	Total =477	X^2	p-value
Hospitals				2.677	0.613
UKMMC	10 (10.6)	84 (89.4)	94		
HPJ	9 (10.0)	81 (90.0)	90		
HSNZ	7 (7.3)	89 (92.7)	96		
HDOK	14 (14.3)	84 (85.7)	98		
SGH	12 (12.1)	87 (87.9)	99		
Age (year)				0.101	0.751
<40	31 (10.5)	263 (89.5)	294		
≥40	21 (11.5)	162 (88.5)	183		
Sex				2.808	0.094
Male	7 (6.5)	101 (93.5)	108		
Female	45 (12.2)	324 (87.8)	369		
Ethnicity				0.127	0.722
Malays	29 (10.5)	248 (89.5)	277		
Non-Malays	23 (11.5)	177 (88.5)	200		
Religion				0.108	0.743
Islam	34 (11.3)	268 (88.7)	302		
Non-Islam	18 (10.3)	157 (89.7)	175		

Career				1.331	0.514
Doctors	17 (10.2)	149 (89.8)	166		
Pharmacists	19 (13.4)	123 (86.6)	142		
Nurses	16 (9.5)	153 (90.5)	169		
Years of working				0.017	0.897
≤10	23 (10.7)	192 (89.3)	215		
>10	29 (11.1)	233 (88.9)	262		
Marital Status				0.234	0.628
Married	32 (10.4)	276 (89.6)	308		
Not married	20 (11.8)	149 (88.2)	169		
Education Level				1.048	0.592
Diploma	13 (8.8)	134 (91.2)	147		
Degree	27 (11.4)	209 (88.6)	236		
Master/PhD	12 (12.8)	82 (87.2)	94		
Income (RM)				0.029	0.864
Low (<4000)	27 (10.7)	226 (89.3)	253		
High (≥4000)	25 (11.2)	199 (88.8)	224		

Table 4.33 shows the association between the use of postnatal care in the last one year and socio-demographic characteristics of the respondents. The finding shows that Malays (20%), Muslims (19.1%) and health professionals who have less than 10 years of working experience (21.4%) were more likely to practice postnatal care during the last one year (p=0.001, p=0.003 and p=0.049 respectively). There was no significant difference in the use of postnatal care in the last one year among the health professionals between hospitals, age, sex, career, education level and income.

Table 4.33 Socio-demographic characteristics and use of postnatal care in the last one year among married female health professionals

Postnatal Care (in the last one year) (Married Female)	Used =39(15.1%) N (%)	Not Used =219(84.9%) N (%) (	Total =258	X^2	p-value
Hospitals				5.341	0.254
UKMMC	6 (11.3)	47 (88.7)	53		
HPJ	13 (24.1)	41 (75.9)	54		
HSNZ	11 (16.4)	56 (83.6)	67		
HDOK	4 (10.3)	35 (89.7)	39		
SGH	5 (11.1)	40 (88.9)	45		
Age (year)				3.025	0.082
<40	26 (18.7)	113 (81.3)	139		
≥40	13 (10.9)	106 (89.1)	119		
Ethnicity				10.111	0.001**
Malays	35 (20.0)	140 (80.0)	175		
Non Malays	4 (4.8)	79 (95.2)	83		
Religion				8.782	0.003**
Islam	36 (19.1)	152 (80.9)	188		
Non Islam	3 (4.3)	67 (95.7)	70		
Career				0.958	0.619
Doctors	13 (18.1)	59 (81.9)	72		
Pharmacists	8 (16.3)	41 (83.7)	49		
Nurses	18 (13.1)	119 (86.9)	137		
Years of working				3.868	0.049*
≤10	18 (21.4)	66 (78.6)	84		

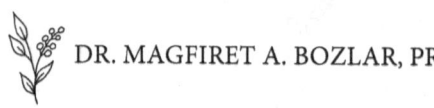

>10	21 (12.1)	153 (87.9)	174		
Education Level				0.38	0.827
Diploma	11 (13.3)	72 (86.7)	83		
Degree	20 (16.4)	102 (83.6)	122		
Master/PhD	8 (15.1)	45 (84.9)	53		
Income (RM)				0.755	0.385
Low (<4000)	22 (17.1)	107 (82.9)	129		
High (≥4000)	17 (13.2)	112 (86.8)	129		

*significant at p<0.05, **significant at p<0.01

Table 4.34 shows the association between the use of other types of T&CM in the last one year and socio-demographic characteristics of the respondents. The finding shows that non-married health professionals were more likely to use other types of T&CM (5.9%) (p=0.04). There was no significant difference in the use of other types of T&CM in the last one year among the health professionals between hospitals, age, sex, ethnicity, religion, career, working experience, education level and income.

Table 4.34 Socio-demographic characteristics and use of other types of T&CM in the last one year among the health professionals

Other Types of T&CM (in the last one year)	Used =17(3.6%) N (%)	Not Used =460(96.4%) N (%)	Total =477	X^2	p-value
Hospitals				6.612	0.158
UKMMC	2 (2.1)	92 (97.9)	94		
HPJ	1 (1.1)	89 (98.9)	90		

PRACTICE OF TRADITIONAL AND COMPLEMENTARY MEDICINE AMONG HEALTH PROFESSIONALS IN MALAYSIA

HSNZ	6 (6.2)	90 (93.8)	96		
HDOK	2 (2.0)	96 (98.0)	98		
SGH	6 (6.1)	93 (93.9)	99		
Age (year)				1.641	0.200
<40	13 (4.4)	281 (95.6)	294		
≥40	4 (2.2)	179 (97.8)	183		
Sex				3.458	0.063
Male	7 (6.5)	101 (93.5)	108		
Female	10 (2.7)	359 (97.3)	369		
Ethnicity				0.319	0.572
Malays	11 (4.0)	266 (96.0)	277		
Non-Malays	6 (3.0)	194 (97.0)	200		
Religion				0.402	0.526
Islam	12 (4.0)	290 (96.0)	302		
Non-Islam	5 (2.9)	170 (97.1)	175		
Career				1.091	0.579
Doctors	7 (4.2)	159 (95.8)	166		
Pharmacists	6 (4.2)	136 (95.8)	142		
Nurses	4 (2.4)	165 (97.6)	169		
Years of working				0.108	0.742
≤10	7 (3.3)	208 (96.7)	215		
>10	10 (3.8)	252 (96.2)	262		
Marital Status				4.217	0.040*
Married	7 (2.3)	301 (97.7)	308		
Not married	10 (5.9)	159 (94.1)	169		
Education Level				0.163	0.922
Diploma	5 (3.4)	142 (96.6)	147		
Degree	8 (3.4)	228 (96.6)	236		
Master/PhD	4 (4.3)	90 (95.7)	94		

Income (RM)				0.237	0.627
Low (<4000)	10 (4.0)	243 (96.0)	253		
High (≥4000)	7 (3.1)	217 (96.9)	224		

*significant at p<0.05

Table 4.35 shows the association between massage referral in the whole life and socio-demographic characteristics of the respondents. The finding shows that health professionals of over 40 years old (41.0%), Malays (36.5%), Muslims (37.1%), nurses (39.1%) and health professionals with working experience of more than 10 years (38.9%) were more likely to do massage referral (p=0.002, p=0.029, p=0.005, p=0.007 and p=0.001 respectively). There was no significant difference between hospitals, sex, marital status, education level, income and referral of massage in whole life among the health professionals.

Table 4.35 Socio-demographic characteristics and referral massage in a whole life among the health professionals

Referral Massage (Whole Life)	Referred =155(32.5%) N (%)	Not Referred =322(67.5%) N (%)	Total =477	X^2	p-value
Hospitals				9.199	0.056
UKMMC	21 (22.3)	73 (77.7)	94		
HPJ	38 (42.2)	52 (57.8)	90		
HSNZ	34 (35.4)	62 (64.6)	96		
HDOK	33 (33.7)	65 (66.3)	98		
SGH	29 (29.3)	70 (70.7)	99		
Age (year)				9.754	0.002**
<40	80 (27.2)	214 (72.8)	294		

PRACTICE OF TRADITIONAL AND COMPLEMENTARY MEDICINE AMONG HEALTH PROFESSIONALS IN MALAYSIA

≥40	75 (41.0)	108 (59.0)	183		
Sex				1.416	0.234
Male	30 (27.8)	78 (72.2)	108		
Female	125 (33.9)	244 (66.1)	369		
Ethnicity				4.74	0.029*
Malays	101 (36.5)	176 (63.5)	277		
Non-Malays	54 (27.0)	146 (73.0)	200		
Religion				7.911	0.005**
Islam	112 (37.1)	190 (62.9)	302		
Non-Islam	43 (24.6)	132 (75.4)	175		
Career				9.992	0.007**
Doctors	57 (34.3)	109 (65.7)	166		
Pharmacists	32 (22.5)	110 (77.5)	142		
Nurses	66 (39.1)	103 (60.9)	169		
Years of working				10.978	0.001**
≤10	53 (24.7)	162 (75.3)	215		
>10	102 (38.9)	160 (61.1)	262		
Marital Status				1.998	0.157
Married	107 (34.7)	201 (65.3)	308		
Not married	48 (28.4)	121 (71.6)	169		
Education Level				0.159	0.923
Diploma	48 (32.7)	99 (67.3)	147		
Degree	75 (31.8)	161 (68.2)	236		
Master/PhD	32 (34)	62 (66.0)	94		
Income (RM)				0.681	0.409
Low (<4000)	78 (30.8)	175 (69.2)	253		
High (≥4000)	77 (34.4)	147 (65.6)	224		

*significant at p<0.05, **significant at p<0.01

Table 4.36 shows the association between acupuncture referral during whole life and socio-demographic characteristics of the respondents. The finding shows that referral of acupuncture was significantly higher at Hospital Putrajaya (20%, p=0.026) and among health professionals aged 40 and above (19.7%, p=0.002), males (20.4%, p=0.02), doctors (23.5%, p<0.001) and high income health professionals (20.1%, p<0.001). There was no significant difference in the referral of acupuncture in whole life among the health professionals between ethnicity, religion, years of working, marital status and education level.

Table 4.36 Socio-demographic characteristics and acupuncture referral in a whole life among the health professionals

Referral Acupuncture (Whole Life)	Referred =65(13.6%) N (%)	Not Referred =412(86.4%) N (%)	Total =477	X^2	p-value
Hospitals				11.022	0.026*
UKMMC	5 (5.3)	89 (94.7)	94		
HPJ	18 (20.0)	72 (80.0)	90		
HSNZ	13 (13.5)	83 (86.5)	96		
HDOK	18 (18.4)	80 (81.6)	98		
SGH	11 (11.1)	88 (88.9)	99		
Age (year)				9.219	0.002**
<40	29 (9,9)	265 (90.1)	294		
≥40	36 (19.7)	147 (80.3)	183		
Sex				5.394	0.020*
Male	22 (20.4)	86 (79.6)	108		
Female	43 (11.7)	326 (88.3)	369		
Ethnicity				1.324	0.250
Malays	42 (15.2)	235 (84.8)	277		

Non-Malays	23 (11.5)	177 (88.5)	200		
Religion				0.622	0.430
Islam	44 (14.6)	258 (85.4)	302		
Non-Islam	21 (12.0)	154 (88.0)	175		
Career				21.063	<0.001***
Doctors	39 (23.5)	127 (76.5)	166		
Pharmacists	12 (8.5)	130 (91.5)	142		
Nurses	14 (8.3)	155 (91.7)	169		
Years of working				2.019	0.155
≤10	24 (11.2)	191 (88.8)	215		
>10	41 (15.6)	221 (84.4)	262		
Marital Status				0.687	0.407
Married	39 (12.7)	269 (87.3)	308		
Not married	26 (15.4)	143 (84.6)	169		
Education Level				1.15	0.563
Diploma	19 (12.9)	128 (87.1)	147		
Degree	30 (12.7)	206 (87.3)	236		
Master/PhD	16 (17.0)	78 (83.0)	94		
Income (RM)				14.985	<0.001***
Low (<4000)	20 (7.9)	233 (92.1)	253		
High (≥4000)	45 (20.1)	179 (79.9)	224		

*significant at p<0.05, **significant at p<0.01, ***significant at p<0.001

Table 4.37 shows the association between herbal medicine referral during whole life and socio-demographic characteristics of the respondents. The finding shows that there was no significant difference in the referral of herbal medicine in the whole life among the health professionals between hospitals, age, sex, ethnicity, religion, career, working experience, marital status, education level and income.

Table 4.37 Socio-demographic characteristics and referral of herbal medicine in a whole life among the health professionals

Referral Herbal Medicine (Whole Life)	Referred= 46(9.6%) N (%)	Not Referred =431(90.4%) N (%)	Total =477	X^2	p-value
Hospitals				3.009	0.556
UKMMC	8 (8.5)	86 (91.5)	94		
HPJ	7 (7.8)	83 (92.2)	90		
HSNZ	8 (8.3)	88 (91.7)	96		
HDOK	9 (9.2)	89 (90.8)	98		
SGH	14 (14.1)	85 (85.9)	99		
Age (year)				1.143	0.285
<40	25 (8.5)	269 (91.5)	294		
≥40	21 (11.5)	162 (88.5)	183		
Sex				0.275	0.600
Male	9 (8.3)	99 (91.7)	108		
Female	37 (10.0)	332 (90.0)	369		
Ethnicity				1.362	0.243
Malays	23 (8.3)	254 (91.7)	277		
Non Malays	23 (11.5)	177 (88.5)	200		
Religion				1.011	0.315
Islam	26 (8.6)	276 (91.4)	302		
Non Islam	20 (11.4)	155 (88.5)	175		
Career				2.66	0.264
Doctors	11 (6.6)	155 (93.4)	166		

Pharmacists	16 (11.3)	126 (88.7)	142			
Nurses	19 (11.2)	150 (88.8)	169			
Years of working					0.052	0.819
≤10	20 (9.3)	195 (90.7)	215			
>10	26 (9.9)	236 (90.1)	262			
Marital Status					2.325	0.127
Married	25 (8.1)	283 (91.9)	308			
Not married	21 (12.4)	148 (87.6)	169			
Education Level					0.767	0.681
Diploma	14 (9.5)	133 (90.5)	147			
Degree	25 (10.6)	211 (89.4)	236			
Master/PhD	7 (7.4)	87 (92.6)	94			
Income(RM)					0.035	0.852
Low(<4000)	25 (9.9)	228 (90.1)	253			
High(≥4000)	21 (9.4)	203 (90.6)	224			

Table 4.38 shows the association between postnatal care referral during whole life and socio-demographic characteristics of the respondents. The finding shows that referral of postnatal care was significantly higher among females (15.7%, p=0.003), Malays (16.6%, p=0.01), Muslims (16.2%, p=0.011), nurses (23.7%, p<0.001), health professionals who have more than 10 years of working experience (16.8%, p=0.011) and married health professionals (18.8%, p<0.001). There was no significant difference in the referral of postnatal care in their whole life among the health professionals between hospitals, age, education level and income.

Table 4.38 Socio-demographic characteristics and postnatal care referral in a whole life among the health professionals

Referral Postnatal Care (Whole Life)	Referred =63(13.2%) N (%)	Not Referred =414(86.8%) N (%)	Total =477	X^2	p-value
Hospitals				6.128	0.190
UKMMC	11(11.7)	83(88.3)	94		
HPJ	16(17.8)	74(82.2)	90		
HSNZ	17(17.7)	79(82.3)	96		
HDOK	11(11.2)	87(88.8)	98		
SGH	8(8.1)	91(91.9)	99		
Age (year)				1.135	0.287
<40	35 (11.9)	25 (88.1)	294		
≥40	28 (15.3)	155 (84.7)	183		
Sex				8.961	0.003**
Male	5 (4.6)	103 (95.4)	108		
Female	58 (15.7)	311 (84.3)	369		
Ethnicity				6.658	0.01*
Malays	46 (16.6)	231 (83.4)	277		
Non-Malays	17 (8.5)	183 (91.5)	200		
Religion				6.539	0.011*
Islam	49 (16.2)	253 (83.8)	302		
Non-Islam	14(8.0)	161 (92.0)	175		
Career				25.004	<0.001***
Doctors	12 (7.2)	154 (92.8)	166		
Pharmacists	11 (7.7)	131 (92.3)	142		
Nurses	40 (23.7)	129 (76.3)	169		
Years of working				6.522	0.011*
≤10	19 (8.8)	196 (91.2)	215		
>10	44 (16.8)	218 (83.2)	262		

Marital Status				23.983	<0.001***
Married	58 (18.8)	250 (81.2)	308		
Not Married	5 (3.0)	164 (97.0)	169		
Education Level				1.574	0.455
Diploma	19 (12.9)	128 (87.1)	147		
Degree	28 (11.9)	208 (88.1)	236		
Master/PhD	16 (17.0)	78 (83.0)	94		
Income (RM)				0.184	0.668
Low (<4000)	35 (13.8)	218 (86.2)	253		
High (≥4000)	28 (12.5)	196 (87.5)	224		

*significant at p<0.05, **significant at p<0.01, ***significant at p<0.001

Table 4.39 shows the association between other types of T&CM referral during whole life and socio-demographic characteristics of the respondents. The finding shows that referral of other types of T&CM was significantly higher among pharmacists (10.6%%, p=0.017). There was no significant difference in the referral of other types of T&CM in their whole life among the health professionals between hospitals, age, sex, ethnicity, religion, working experience, marital status, education level and income.

Table 4.39 Socio-demographic characteristics and referral of other types of T&CM during whole life among the health professionals

Referral Other Types of T&CM (Whole Life)	Referred =28(5.9%) N (%)	Not Referred =449(94.1%) N (%)	Total =477	X^2	p-value
Hospitals				1.423	0.840
UKMMC	4 (4.3)	90 (95.7)	94		
HPJ	5 (5.6)	85 (94.4)	90		
HSNZ	5 (5.2)	91 (94.8)	96		
HDOK	6 (6.1)	92 (93.9)	98		
SGH	8 (8.1)	91 (91.9)	99		
Age (year)				2.247	0.134
<40	21 (7.1)	273 (92.9)	294		
≥40	7 (3.8)	176 (96.2)	183		
Sex				1.533	0.216
Male	9 (8.3)	99 (91.7)	108		
Female	19 (5.1)	350 (94.9)	369		
Ethnicity				0.247	0.619
Malays	15 (5.4)	262 (94.6)	277		
Non-Malays	13 (6.5)	187 (93.5)	200		
Religion				0.086	0.769
Islam	17 (5.6)	285 (94.4)	302		
Not-Islam	11 (6.3)	164 (93.7)	175		
Career				8.103	0.017*
Doctors	6 (3.6)	160 (96.4)	166		
Pharmacists	15 (10.6)	127 (89.4)	142		
Nurses	7 (4.1)	162 (95.9)	169		
Years of working				0.868	0.352
≤10	15 (7.0)	200 (93.0)	215		
>10	13 (5.0)	249 (95.0)	262		
Marital Status				2.760	0.097
Married	14 (4.5)	294 (95.5)	308		

PRACTICE OF TRADITIONAL AND COMPLEMENTARY MEDICINE AMONG HEALTH PROFESSIONALS IN MALAYSIA

Not married	14 (8.3)	155 (91.7)	169		
Education Level				3.008	0.222
Diploma	8 (5.4)	139 (94.6)	147		
Degree	11 (4.7)	225 (95.3)	236		
Master/PhD	9 (9.6)	85 (90.4)	94		
Income (RM)				0.703	0.402
Low (<4000)	17 (6.7)	236 (93.3)	253		
High (≥4000)	11 (4.9)	213 (95.1)	224		

*significant at p<0.05

Table 4.40 shows the association between referral massage in the last one year and socio-demographic characteristics of the respondents. The finding shows that there was no significant difference in the massage referral in the last one year among the health professionals between hospitals, age, sex, ethnicity, religion, career, working experience, marital status, education level and income.

Table 4.40 Socio-demographic characteristics and massage referral in the last one year among health professionals

Massage Referral (in the last one year)	Referred =78(16.4%) N (%)	Not Referred =399(83.6%) N (%)	Total =477	X^2	p-value
Hospitals				4.831	0.305
UKMMC	9 (9.6)	85 (90.4)	94		
HPJ	18 (20.0)	72 (80.0)	90		
HSNZ	18 (18.8)	78 (81.2)	96		
HDOK	18 (18.4)	80 (81.6)	98		
SGH	15 (15.2)	84 (84.8)	99		

Age (year)				3.245	0.072
<40	41 (13.9)	253 (86.1)	294		
≥40	37 (20.2)	146 (79.8)	183		
Sex				0.976	0.323
Male	21 (19.4)	87 (80.6)	108		
Female	57 (15.4)	312 (84.6)	369		
Ethnicity				0.864	0.353
Malay	49 (17.7)	228 (82.3)	277		
Non Malay	29 (14.5)	171 (85.5)	200		
Religion				0.863	0.353
Islam	53 (17.5)	249 (82.5)	302		
Non Islam	25 (14.3)	150 (85.7)	175		
Career				2.004	0.367
Doctors	30 (18.1)	136 (81.9)	166		
Pharmacists	18 (12.7)	124 (87.3)	142		
Nurses	30 (17.8)	139 (82.2)	169		
Years of working				1.647	0.199
≤10	30 (14.0)	185 (86.0)	215		
>10	48 (18.3)	214 (81.7)	262		
Marital Status				0.465	0.495
Married	53 (17.2)	255 (82.8)	308		
Not married	25 (14.8)	144 (85.2)	169		
Education Level				0.271	0.873
Diploma	23 (15.6)	124 (84.4)	147		
Degree	38 (16.1)	198 (83.9)	236		
Master/PhD	17 (18.1)	77 (81.9)	94		
Income (RM)				1.775	0.183
Low (<4000)	36 (14.2)	217 (85.8)	253		
High (≥4000)	42 (18.8)	182 (81.2)	224		

PRACTICE OF TRADITIONAL AND COMPLEMENTARY MEDICINE AMONG HEALTH PROFESSIONALS IN MALAYSIA

Table 4.41 shows the association between acupuncture referral in the last one year and socio-demographic characteristic of the respondents. The finding shows that referral acupuncture was significantly higher among male health professionals (14.8%%, p=0.009), doctors (16.9%, p<0.001) and high income health professionals (14.3%, p<0.001). There was no significant difference in the acupuncture referral in the last one year among the health professionals between hospitals, age, ethnicity, religion, working experience, marital status, education level and income.

Table 4.41 Socio-demographic characteristics and acupuncture referral in the last one year among the health professionals

Acupuncture Referral (in the last one year)	Referred =41(8.6%) N (%)	Not Referred =436(91.4%) N (%)	Total =477	X^2	p-value
Hospitals				5.421	0.247
UKMMC	3 (3.2)	91 (96.8)	94		
HPJ	9 (10.0)	81 (90.0)	90		
HSNZ	8 (8.3)	88 (91.7)	96		
HDOK	12 (12.2)	86 (87.8)	98		
SGH	9 (9.1)	90 (90.9)	99		
Age (year)				3.135	0.077
<40	20 (6.8)	274 (93.2)	294		
≥40	21 (11.5)	162 (88.5)	183		
Sex				6.874	0.009**
Male	16 (14.8)	92 (85.2)	108		
Female	25 (6.8)	344 (93.2)	369		
Ethnicity				0.526	0.468

Malays	26 (9.4)	251 (90.6)	277		
Non Malays	15 (7.5)	185 (92.5)	200		
Religion				0.637	0.959
Islam	27 (8.9)	275 (91.1)	302		
Non Islam	8 (7.7)	96 (92.3)	104		
Career				22.362	<0.001***
Doctors	28 (16.9)	138 (83.1)	166		
Pharmacists	7 (4.9)	135 (95.1)	142		
Nurses	6 (3.6)	163 (96.4)	169		
Years of working				0.663	0.416
≤10	16 (7.4)	199 (92.6)	215		
>10	25 (9.5)	237 (90.5)	262		
Marital Status				0.714	0.398
Married	24 (7.8)	284 (92.2)	308		
Not married	17 (10.1)	152 (89.9)	169		
Education Level				0.735	0.692
Diploma	11 (7.5)	136 (92.5)	147		
Degree	20 (8.5)	216 (91.5)	236		
Master/PhD	10 (10.6)	84 (89.4)	94		
Income (RM)				17.406	<0.001***
Low (<4000)	9 (3.6)	244 (96.4)	253		
High (≥4000)	32 (14.3)	192 (85.7)	224		

**significant at p<0.01, ***significant at p<0.001

Table 4.42 shows the association between herbal medicine referral in the last one year and socio-demographic characteristics of the respondents. The finding shows that there was no significant difference in the herbal medicine referral in the last one year among the health professionals between socio-demographic factors such ass hospitals, age, ethnicity, religion, working experience, marital status, education level and income.

Table 4.42 Socio-demographic characteristics and herbal medicine referral in the last one year among the health professionals

Herbal Medicine Referral (in the last one year)	Referred =23(4.8%) N (%)	Not Referred =454(95.2%) N (%)	Total =477	X²	p-value
Hospitals				4.055	0.399
UKMMC	5 (5.3)	89 (94.7)	94		
HPJ	4 (4.4)	86 (95.6)	90		
HSNZ	2 (2.1)	94 (97.9)	96		
HDOK	4 (4.1)	94 (95.9)	98		
SGH	8 (8.1)	91 (91.9)	99		
Age (year)				1.949	0.163
<40	11 (3.7)	283 (96.3)	294		
≥40	12 (6.6)	171 (93.4)	183		
Sex				0.011	0.916
Male	5 (4.6)	103 (95.4)	108		
Female	18 (4.9)	351 (95.1)	369		
Ethnicity				0.024	0.877
Malays	13 (4.7)	264 (95.3)	277		
Non-Malays	10 (5.0)	190 (95.0)	200		
Religion				0.038	0.846
Islam	15 (5.0)	287 (95.0)	302		
Non-Islam	8 (4.6)	167 (95.4)	175		
Career				3.258	0.196

Doctors	4 (2.4)	162 (97.6)	166		
Pharmacists	9 (6.3)	133 (93.7)	142		
Nurses	10 (5.9)	159 (94.1)	169		
Years of working				0.345	0.557
≤10	9 (4.2)	206 (95.8)	215		
>10	14 (5.3)	248 (94.7)	262		
Marital Status				1.623	0.203
Married	12 (3.9)	296 (96.1)	308		
Not married	11 (6.5)	158 (93.5)	157		
Education Level				3.611	0.164
Diploma	3 (2.0)	144 (98.0)	147		
Degree	14 (5.9)	222 (94.1)	236		
Master/PhD	6 (6.4)	88 (93.6)	94		
Income (RM)				0.007	0.932
Low (<4000)	12 (4.7)	241 (95.3)	253		
High(≥4000)	11 (4.9)	231 (95.1)	224		

Table 4.43 shows the association between postnatal care referral in the last one year and socio-demographic characteristic of the respondents. The finding shows that married health professionals were more likely to refer postnatal care to their patients and family (5.8%, p=0.038).

Table 4.43 Socio-demographic characteristics and postnatal care referral in the last one year among the health professionals

PRACTICE OF TRADITIONAL AND COMPLEMENTARY MEDICINE AMONG HEALTH PROFESSIONALS IN MALAYSIA

Referral Postnatal Care (in the last one year)	Referred =21(4.4%) N (%)	Not Referred =456(95.6%) N (%)	Total =477	X²	p-value
Hospitals				4.436	0.350
UKMMC	2 (2.1)	92 (97.9)	94		
HPJ	3 (3.3)	87 (96.7)	90		
HSNZ	7 (7.3)	89 (92.7)	96		
HDOK	6 (6.1)	92 (93.9)	98		
SGH	3 (3.0)	96 (97.0)	99		
Age (year)				0.891	0.345
<40	15 (5.1)	279 (94.9)	294		
≥40	6 (3.3)	177 (96.7)	183		
Sex				0.162	0.687
Male	4 (3.7)	104 (96.3)	108		
Female	17 (4.6)	352 (95.4)	369		
Ethnicity				0.667	0.414
Malays	14 (5.1)	263 (94.9)	277		
Non-Malays	7 (3.5)	193 (96.5)	200		
Religion				0.623	0.430
Islam	15 (5.0)	287 (95.0)	302		
Non-Islam	6 (3.4)	169 (96.6)	175		
Career				2.806	0.246
Doctors	5 (3.0)	161 (97.0)	166		
Pharmacists	5 (3.5)	137 (96.5)	142		
Nurses	11 (6.5)	158 (93.5)	169		
Years of working				0.432	0.511
≤10	8 (3.7)	207 (96.3)	215		
>10	13 (5)	249 (95)	262		
Marital Status				4.293	0.038*

Married	18 (5.8)	290 (94.2)	308		
Not Married	3 (1.8)	166 (98.2)	169		
Education Level				1.436	0.488
Diploma	4 (2.7)	143 (97.3)	147		
Degree	12 (5.1)	224 (94.9)	236		
Master/PhD	5 (5.3)	89 (94.7)	94		
Income (RM)				0.148	0.700
Low (<4000)	12 (4.7)	241 (95.3)	253		
High (≥4000)	9 (4)	215 (96)	224		

*significant at $p<0.05$

Table 4.44 shows the association between referral of other types of T&CM in the last one year and socio-demographic characteristics of the respondents. The finding shows that there was no significant difference in the referral of other types of T&CM in the last one year among the health professionals between socio-demographic characteristics of the respondents such as hospitals, age, sex, ethnicity, religion, career, working experience, marital status, education level and income.

Table 4.44 Socio-demographic characteristics and referral other types of T&CM in the last one year among the health professionals

Referral Others Types of T&CM (in the last one year)	Referred =14(3.0%) N (%)	Not Referred =463(97%) N (%)	Total =477	X^2	P Value
Hospitals				2.333	0.675

PRACTICE OF TRADITIONAL AND COMPLEMENTARY MEDICINE AMONG HEALTH PROFESSIONALS IN MALAYSIA

UKMMC	3 (3.2)	91 (96.8)	94		
HPJ	2 (2.2)	88 (97.8)	90		
HSNZ	2 (2.1)	94 (97.9)	96		
HDOK	5 (5.1)	93 (94.9)	98		
SGH	2 (2.0)	97 (98.0)	99		
Age (year)				0.123	0.726
<40	8 (2.7)	286 (97.3)	294		
≥40	6 (3.3)	177 (96.7)	183		
Sex				1.407	0.236
Male	5 (4.6)	103 (95.4)	108		
Female	9 (2.4)	360 (97.6)	369		
Male	5 (4.6)	103 (95.4)	108		
Female	9 (2.4)	360 (97.6)	369		
Ethnicity				0.386	0.534
Malays	7 (2.5)	270 (97.5)	277		
Non Malays	7 (3.5)	193 (96.5)	200		
Religion				0.236	0.627
Islam	8 (2.6)	294 (97.4)	302		
Non Islam	6 (3.4)	169 (96.6)	175		
Career				1.571	0.456
Doctors	3 (1.8)	163 (98.2)	166		
Pharmacists	6 (4.2)	136 (95.8)	142		
Nurses	5 (3.0)	164 (97.0)	169		
Years of working				0.141	0.707
≤10	7 (3.3)	208 (96.7)	215		
>10	7 (2.7)	255 (97.3)	262		
Marital Status				0.348	0.555
Married	8 (2.6)	30 (97.4)	308		
Not married	6 (3.6)	163 (96.4)	169		
Education Level				2.451	0.294

Diploma	4 (2.7)	143 (97.3)	147		
Degree	5 (2.1)	231 (97.9)	236		
Master/PhD	5 (5.3)	89 (94.7)	94		
Income (RM)				0.732	0.392
Low (<4000)	9 (3.6)	244 (96.4)	253		
High(≥4000)	5 (2.2)	219 (97.8)	224		

Table 4.45 shows the association between knowledge regarding T&CM and socio-demographic characteristic of the respondents. The finding shows that knowledge regarding T&CM was significantly higher in Hospital Duchess of Kent (52%, p=0.001), among non-Malays (44%, p=0.047), pharmacists (47.2%, p=0.03). There were no significant difference in the knowledge regarding T&CM among the health professionals between age, sex, religion, working experience, marital status, education level and income

Table 4.45 Relationship between socio-demographic factors and knowledge regarding T&CM among the health professionals

Knowledge	Good Knowledge =185(38.8%) N (%)	Poor Knowledge =292 (61.2%) N (%)	Total =477	X^2	p-value
Hospitals				18.971	0.001**
UKMMC	24 (25.5)	70 (74.5)	94		
HPJ	43 (47.8)	47 (52.2)	90		
HSNZ	34 (35.4)	62 (64.6)	96		
HDOK	51 (52.0)	47 (48.0)	98		
SGH	33 (33.3)	66 (66.7)	99		

PRACTICE OF TRADITIONAL AND COMPLEMENTARY MEDICINE AMONG HEALTH PROFESSIONALS IN MALAYSIA

Age (year)				1.356	0.244
<40	108 (36.7)	186 (63.3)	294		
≥40	77 (42.1)	106 (57.9)	183		
Sex				0.040	0.842
Male	41 (38.0)	67 (62.0)	108		
Female	144 (39.0)	225 (61.0)	369		
Ethnicity				3.947	0.047*
Malays	97 (35.0)	180 (65.0)	277		
Non Malays	88 (44.0)	112 (56.0)	200		
Religion				1.428	0.232
Islam	111 (36.8)	191 (63.2)	302		
Non Islam	74 (42.3)	101 (57.7)	175		
Career				7.013	0.030*
Doctors	54 (32.5)	112 (67.5)	166		
Pharmacists	67 (47.2)	75 (52.8)	142		
Nurses	64 (37.9)	105 (62.1)	169		
Years of working				0.005	0.942
≤10	83 (38.6)	132 (61.4)	215		
>10	102 (38.9)	160 (61.1)	262		
Marital Status				1.653	0.198
Married	126 (40.9)	182 (59.1)	308		
Not married	59 (34.9)	110 (65.1)	169		
Education				1.799	0.407
Diploma	59 (40.1)	88 (59.9)	147		
Degree	85 (36.0)	151 (64.0)	236		
Master/PhD	41 (43.6)	53 (56.4)	94		
Income(RM)				0.001	0.981
Low(<4000)	98 (38.7)	155 (61.3)	253		
High(≥4000)	87 (38.8)	137 (61.2)	224		

*significant at p<0.05, **significant at p<0.01

Table 4.46 shows the association between attitudes towards T&CM and socio-demographic characteristic of the respondents. The finding shows that a positive attitude towards T&CM was high among health professionals in Hospital Sultanah NurZahirah (78.1%, p<0.001), females (69.1%, p=0.002), Malays (70.8%, p=0.004), Muslims (70.5%, p=0.002), nurses (76.3%, p<0.001), health professionals who had more than 10 years' working experience (70.2%, p=0.015), health professionals who gained diploma (74.8%, p=0.006) and the low-income health professionals (70.8%, p=0.009). There was no significant difference in the attitude towards T&CM between age and marital status.

Table 4.46 Relationship between socio-demographic factors and attitude towards T&CM among the health professionals

Attitude	Positive attitude =312(65.4%) N (%)	Negative attitude =165(34.6%) N (%)	Total =477	X^2	p-value
Hospitals				20.668	<0.001***
UKMMC	46 (48.9)	48 (51.1)	94		
HPJ	63 (70.0)	27 (30.0)	90		
HSNZ	75 (78.1)	21 (21.9)	96		
HDOK	68 (69.4)	30 (30.6)	98		
SGH	60 (60.6)	39 (39.4)	99		
Age (year)				3.39	0.066
<40	183 (62.2)	111 (37.8)	294		
≥40	129 (70.5)	54 (29.5)	183		
Sex				9.844	0.002**
Male	57 (52.8)	51 (47.1)	108		
Female	255 (69.1)	114 (30.9)	369		

PRACTICE OF TRADITIONAL AND COMPLEMENTARY MEDICINE AMONG HEALTH PROFESSIONALS IN MALAYSIA

Ethnicity				8.355	0.004**
Malays	196 (70.8)	81 (29.2)	277		
Non Malays	116 (58.0)	84 (42.0)	200		
Religion				9.541	0.002**
Islam	213 (70.5)	89 (29.5)	302		
Non Islam	99 (56.6)	76 (43.4)	175		
Career				26.161	<0.001***
Doctors	84 (50.6)	82 (49.4)	166		
Pharmacists	99 (69.7)	43 (30.3)	142		
Nurses	129 (76.3)	40 (23.7)	169		
Years of working				5.969	0.015*
≤10	128 (59.5)	87 (40.5)	215		
>10	184 (70.2)	78 (29.8)	262		
Marital Status				0.835	0.361
Married	206 (66.9)	102 (33.1)	308		
Not married	106 (62.7)	63 (37.3)	169		
Education Level				10.296	0.006**
Diploma	110 (74.8)	37 (25.2)	147		
Degree	139 (58.9)	97 (41.1)	236		
Master/PhD	63 (67.0)	31 (33)	94		
Income (RM)				6.796	0.009**
Low (<4000)	179 (70.8)	74 (29.2)	253		
High (≥4000)	133 (59.4)	91 (40.6)	224		

*significant at p<0.05, **significant at p<0.01, ***significant at p<0.001

Table 4.47 shows the association between perception regarding education and socio-demographic characteristics of the respondents. The finding shows that positive perception regarding education in T&CM among health professionals was higher among females (88.1%, p=0.002) and pharmacists (93.7%, p<0.001). There was no significant difference in the perception regarding education in T&CM between hospital, age, ethnicity, religion, years of working, marital status, education level and income.

Table 4.47 Relationship between socio-demographic factors and perception regarding education in T&CM among the health professionals

Perception	Positive perception =407(85.0%) N (%)	Negative perception =70(15.0%) N (%)	Total =477	X^2	p-value
Hospitals				3.262	0.515
UKMMC	77 (81.9)	17 (18.1)	94		
HPJ	77 (85.6)	13 (14.4)	90		
HSNZ	87 (90.6)	9 (9.4)	96		
HDOK	82 (83.7)	16 (16.3)	98		
SGH	84 (84.8)	15 (15.2)	99		
Age (year)				0.244	0.622
<40	249 (84.7)	45 (15.3)	294		
≥40	158 (86.3)	25 (13.7)	183		
Sex				9.85	0.002**
Male	82 (75.9)	26 (24.1)	108		
Female	325 (88.1)	44 (11.9)	369		
Ethnicity				0.483	0.487
Malays	239 (86.3)	38 (13.7)	277		
No- Malays	168 (84.0)	32 (16.0)	200		
Religion				2.039	0.153
Islam	263 (87.1)	39 (12.9)	302		

PRACTICE OF TRADITIONAL AND COMPLEMENTARY MEDICINE AMONG HEALTH PROFESSIONALS IN MALAYSIA

Non Islam	144 (82.3)	31 (17.7)	175		
Career				16.986	<0.001***
Doctors	128 (77.1)	38 (22.9)	166		
Pharmacists	133 (93.7)	9 (6.3)	142		
Nurses	146 (86.4)	23 (13.6)	169		
Years of working				0.014	0.907
≤10	183 (85.1)	32 (14.9)	215		
>10	224 (85.5)	38 (14.5)	262		
Marital Status				0.237	0.626
Married	261 (84.7)	47 (15.3)	308		
Not married	146 (86.4)	23 (13.6)	169		
Education Level				2.209	0.331
Diploma	129 (87.8)	18 (12.2)	147		
Degree	202 (85.6)	34 (14.4)	236		
Master/PhD	76 (80.9)	18 (19.1)	94		
Income (RM)				2.524	0.112
Low (<4000)	222 (87.7)	31 (12.3)	253		
High (≥4000)	185 (82.6)	39 (17.4)	224		

**significant at $p<0.01$, ***significant at $p<0.001$

Table 4.48 shows the association between knowledge on T&CM, attitude towards T&CM, perception regarding education in T&CM and use of T&CM. The finding shows that health professionals who have positive attitude towards T&CM (51.9%) are more likely to use T&CM in their life ($p=0.001$).

Table 4.48 Relationship between knowledge on T&CM, attitude regarding T&CM and perception of education in T&CM and the use of T&CM

	Used=221(46.3%) N (%)	Not Used =256(53.7%) N (%)	Total =477	X^2	p-value
Knowledge					
Good	96 (51.9)	89 (48.1)	185	3.758	0.053
Poor	125 (42.8)	167 (57.2)	292		
Attitude					
Positive	162 (51.9)	150 (48.1)	312	11.342	0.001**
Negative	59 (35.8)	106 (64.2)	165		
Perception					
Positive	193 (47.4)	214 (52.6)	407	1.323	0.250
Negative	28 (40.0)	42 (60.0)	70		

**significant at p<0.01

MULTIVARIABLE LOGISTIC REGRESSION ANALYSIS TO PREDICT THE USE AND REFERRAL TO T&CM AMONG HEALTH PROFESSIONALS

Multivariable logistic regression analysis was used to evaluate the relationships of all independent explanatory factors with the dichotomous outcome variables of use and referral of T&CM in a whole life, in the last one year, referral in a whole life and in the last one year. Therefore, the confounding effects were eliminated, allowing for evaluation of the independent effect of each independent variable on the outcome measure. All statistically significant variables were used for further analysis in order to develop the best mode in terms of association and significance.

Simple logistic regression (SLR) models were run for all dependent variables of use of T&CM in the whole life, in the last one year, referral in the whole life and in the last one year as a preliminary step before subjecting them to the final logistic regression model.

Likelihood ratio (LR) test values were calculated for all independent factors, with one or two levels denoted by a superscript (^{a}), while Wald tests values were considered for those variables with more than two levels denoted by a superscript (^{b}). P-values were considered and denoted according to the selected test statistics, whether LR test (^{a}) or Wald tests (^{b}).

Multivariate Logistic Regression for the Practice of T&CM

Table 4.49 shows the final logistic regression model for the use of T&CM in a whole life, the last one year, referred in a whole life and in the last one year with other determinant variables, with simultaneous adjustment for hospitals, age, sex, ethnicity, religion, career, years of working, marital status, education level and income.

The final logistic regression model revealed that female respondents were 1.5 times more likely to use T&CM as compared to males. Married health professionals were 2.1 times more likely to use T&CM than non-married health professionals. High income health professionals were less likely to use T&CM (AOR=0.664) as compared with the low-income health professionals. Health professionals who had positive attitude towards T&CM were 1.7 times more likely to use T&CM in their whole life.

Female health professionals were 1.9 times more likely to use T&CM compared with males. Married health professionals were 1.5 times more likely to use T&CM compared with non-married health professionals. Health professionals who had positive attitude towards T&CM were 2.2 times more likely to use T&CM in the last one year.

Muslim health professionals were 1.4 times more likely to opt for referral T&CM compared with non-Muslims. Health professionals who had more than 10 years of service were 1.7 times more likely to choose referral T&CM than the health professionals who had less than 10 years of working experience. Health professionals who had good knowledge of T&CM were 1.6 times more likely to choose referral T&CM than the health professionals who had poor knowledge regarding T&CM. Health professionals who had positive attitude were 2.0 times more likely to refer to T&CM than the health professionals who had negative attitude towards T&CM in their life.

Female health professionals were 0.437 times less likely to choose referral T&CM than males. High income health professionals were 1.516 times more likely to choose referral T&CM than low income health professionals. Health professionals who had positive attitude were 2.814 times more likely to choose referral T&CM than the health professionals who had negative attitude towards T&CM in the last one year.

Table 4.49 Multivariable logistic regression to determine factors associated with the use and referral of T&CM

Independent Variable		AOR	95%CI AOR	X²(df)ᵃ	p-valueᵃ
Use of T&CM (Whole life)					
Sex	Male	1			
	Female	1.506	0.945-2.4	2.966(1)	0.085
Marital Status	Married	2.111	1.398-3.18	12.603 (1)	<0.001***
	Not married	1			
Income	Low	1			
	High	0.664	0.448-0.98	4.165(1)	0.041*
Attitude	Negative	1			
	Positive	1.745	1.169-2.60	7.423(1)	0.006**
Use of T&CM in 1 year					
Sex	Male	1			
	Female	1.885	1.113-3.19	5.565(1)	0.018*
Marital Status	Married	1.478	0.966-2.26	3.241(1)	0.072
	Not married	1			
Attitude	Negative	1			
	Positive	2.152	1.381-3.35	11.464(1)	0.001**
Referred T&CM in life time					

Religion	Islam	1.43	0.96-2.131	3.091(1)	0.079
	Non Islam	1			
Years of working	≤10	1			
	>10	1.659	1.134-2.42	6.787(1)	0.009**
Knowledge	Poor	1			
	Good	1.620	1.32-.1053	10.433(1)	0.010*
Attitude	Negative	1			
	Positive	2.024	1.401-3.26	12.401(1)	<0.001***
Referred T&CM in I year					
Sex	Male	1			
	Female	0.437	0.268-0.71	10.953 (1)	0.001**
Income	Low	1			
	High	1.516	0.983-2.33	3.541(1)	0.060
Attitude	Negative	1			
	Positive	2.814	1.696-4.66	16.043(1)	<0.001***

Adj. OR = Adjusted Odds Ratio; [a] Likelihood Ratio (LR) test; [b] Wald test
*significant at p<0.05, **significant at p<0.01, ***significant at p<0.001

Multivariable Logistic Regression for Modalities of T&CM

Table 4.50 displays the final logistic regression model for T&CM modalities with other determinant variables. The final logistic regression model revealed that the staff at Hospital Duchess of Kent were 1.7 times more likely to use massage therapies compared to that of UKMMC, but at the other three hospitals were less likely to use massage as compared to UKMMC. Married health professionals were 2.4 times more likely to use massage therapies compared to the non-married health professionals. Health professionals who had positive attitude were 2.2 times more likely to use massage than those who had negative attitude towards T&CM in their whole life. Muslims were less likely (AOR=0.21) to use acupuncture compared to non-Muslims.

Health professionals who had good knowledge of T&CM were 1.7 times more likely to use herbal medicine compared to the health professionals who had poor knowledge. Health professionals who had positive attitude were 1.7 times more likely to use herbal medicine compared to the health professionals who had negative attitude towards T&CM in their whole life.

The health professionals at Hospital Duchess of Kent (HDOK) were 4.0 times, Hospital Putrajaya (HPJ) 3.6 times, Sarawak General Hospital (SGH) 2.7 times and Hospital Sultanah NurZahirah (HSNZ) 2.7 times more likely to use postnatal care than those at UKMMC. Malays were 2.3 times more likely to use postnatal care compared with non-Malays in their whole life.

Health professionals at the age of 40 and above were less likely (AOR=0.417) to use other types of T&CM than those less than 40 years old. Female health professionals were less likely (AOR=0.396) to use other types of T&CM than males.

Table 4.50 Multivariate logistic regression to determine modalities of T&CM associated with the use of T&CM in the whole life among the health professionals

Independent Variable		AOR	95% CI	X^2 df	p-value@
Massage					
Hospital Name				11.857 (4)	0.018*
	UKMMC	1			
	HPJ	0.732	0.348-1.536	0.683(1)	0.409
	HSNZ	0.684	0.331-1.413	1.054 (1)	0.305
	HDOK	1.727	0.871-3.425	2.45(1)	0.118
	SGH	0.589	0.274-1.267	1.832(1)	0.176
Marital status	Married	2.414	1.414-4.12	10.428 (1)	0.001**
	Not married	1			
Attitude	Negative	1			
	Positive	2.240	1.31-3.828	8.692(1)	0.003**
Acupuncture					
Religion	Islam	0.210	0.73-0.599	8.513(1)	0.004**
	Non Islam	1			
Herbal medicine					
Knowledge	Poor	1			

PRACTICE OF TRADITIONAL AND COMPLEMENTARY MEDICINE AMONG HEALTH PROFESSIONALS IN MALAYSIA

	Good	1.720	1.056-2.801	4.749(1)	0.029*
Attitude	Negative	1			
	Positive	1.673	0.953-2.939	3.211(1)	0.073
Postnatal care					
Hospital Name				9.877 (4)	0.043*
	UKMMC	1			
	HPJ	3.619	1.505-8.703	8.465(1)	0.004**
	HSNZ	2.676	1.144-6.259	5.156(1)	0.023*
	HDOK	3.975	1.35-11.629	6.351(1)	0.548
	SGH	2.709	0.96-7.64	3.547(1)	0.060
Ethnicity	Malay	2.299	1.066-4.957	4.508(1)	0.034*
	Non Malay	1			
Other types of T&CM treatments					
Age (years)				12.72(3)	0.005**
	<40	1			
	≥40	0.417	0.152-1.142	2.893(1)	0.089
Sex	Male	1			
	Female	0.396	0.17-0.922	4.613(1)	0.032**

Adj. OR = Adjusted Odds Ratio; [a] Likelihood Ratio (LR) test; [b] Wald test
*significant at p<0.05, **significant at p<0.01

Table 4.51 shows the final logistic regression model for modalities of using T&CM in the last one year with other determinant variables. The final logistic regression model revealed that nurses were 2.4 times more likely to use massage therapy as compared to doctors. On the contrary, pharmacists were less likely (AOR=0.801) to use massage. Respondents who had high income were 1.7 times more likely to use massage in the last one year.

Muslims were less likely (AOR=0.197) to use acupuncture compared with the non-Muslims, and married health professionals were less likely (AOR=0.335) less likely to use acupuncture than the non-married health professionals in the last one year.

Health professionals who had good knowledge of T&CM were 1.9 times more likely to use herbal medicine than those with poor knowledge. Health professionals who had positive attitude were 3.0 times more likely to use herbal medicine than those who had negative attitude in the last one year.

Malays were 5.9 times more likely to use postnatal care than the non-Malays. Health professionals who had less than 10 years of working experience were 2.3 times more likely to use postnatal care than those who had 10 or more years of working experience. The health professionals who had positive perception in education were 2.6 times more likely to use postnatal care in the last one year.

However, HSNZ was 4.5 times and SGH 2.8 times more likely to use other types of T&CM than UKMMC, and HDOK

(AOR=0.769) and HPJ were (AOR=0.572) times less likely to use other types of T&CM in the last one year.

Health professionals of 40 years old and above were 4.5 times more likely to use other types of T&CM than those below 40 years old. Male health professionals were 3.8 times more likely to use other types of T&CM than females. The health professionals who had 10 years or more of working experience were 4.4 times more likely to use other types of T&CM than those who had less than 10 years of working experience. Non-married health professionals were 4.4 times more likely to use other types of T&CM than those the health professionals in the last one year.

Table 4.51 Multivariable logistic regression to determine modalities of T&CM associated with the use of T&CM in the last one year among the health professionals

Independent Variable		AOR	95% CI	X^2 df	p-value@
Massage					
Career				10.821(1)	0.004**
	Doctor	1			
	Pharmacist	0.801	0.354-1.808	0.286(1)	0.593
	Nurse	2.402	1.19-4.848	5.985(1)	0.014*
Income (RM)	Low (>4000)	1			
	High (≤4000)	1.681	0.906-3.116	2.716(1)	0.099
Acupuncture					
Religion	Islam	0.197	0.052-0.749	5.686(1)	0.017*

	Non Islam	1			
Marital Status	Married	0.335	0.098-1.144	3.047(1)	0.081
	Not married	1			
Herbal Medicine					
Knowledge	Poor	1			
	Good	1.921	1.036-3.565	4.289(1)	0.038*
Attitude	Negative	1			
	Positive	2.956	1.254-6.971	6.131(1)	0.013*
Postnatal Care					
Ethnicity	Malay	5.876	1.958-17.63	9.975(1)	0.002**
	Non Malay	1			
Years of working	≤10	1			
	>10	0.434	0.209-0.901	5.014(1)	0.025*
Perception in education					
	Negative	1			
	Positive	0.381	0.153-0.947	4.311(1)	0.038*
Other types of T&CM treatment					
Hospital				7.397(4)	0.116
	UKMMC	1			
	HPJ	0.572	0.5-6.61	0.2(1)	0.655
	HSNZ	4.463	0.82-24.205	3.007 (1)	0.083
	HDOK	0.769	0.103-5.751	0.065(1)	0.798
	SGH	2.772	0.526-14.6	1.447(1)	0.229
Age (year)	<40	1			

PRACTICE OF TRADITIONAL AND COMPLEMENTARY MEDICINE AMONG HEALTH PROFESSIONALS IN MALAYSIA

	≥40	0.223	0.057-0.878	4.602(1)	0.032*
Sex	Male	1			
	Female	0.264	0.088-0.789	5.689 (1)	0.017*
Year of working	≤10	1			
	>10	4.411	1.198-16.24	4.981(1)	0.026*
Marital Status	Married	0.256	0.084-0.781	5.732(1)	0.017*
	Not married	1			

Adj. OR = Adjusted odds ratio; [a] Likelihood Ratio (LR) test; [b] Wald test
*significant at $p<0.05$, **significant at $p<0.01$

Table 4.52 displays the final logistic regression model for massage referral in a whole life with other determinant variables. The final logistic regression model revealed that health professionals at the age of 40 years old and above were 1.7 times more likely to refer to T&CM compared to health professionals below 40 years old. Muslims were 1.6 times more likely to refer to T&CM compared with non-Muslims. Health professionals who had positive attitude were 1.7 times more likely to refer to massage than who had negative attitude towards T&CM in their whole life.

HPJ was 4.9 times, HDOK was 4.1 times, HSNZ was 3.6 times and SGH was 2.5 times more likely to refer to acupuncture than UKMMC. Health professionals of the age of 40 and above were 2.0 times more likely to refer to acupuncture than those below the age of 40 in their whole life. Doctors were 3 times more likely to refer to acupuncture than pharmacists, and 2.8 times more likely than nurses.

Married health professionals were 2.1 times more likely to refer to acupuncture than non-married health professionals. High income health professionals were 2.6 times more likely to refer to acupuncture than low- income health professionals. Health professionals who had good knowledge regarding acupuncture were 1.9 times more likely to refer to acupuncture than those with poor knowledge. Health professionals who had positive attitude were 2,0 times more likely to refer to acupuncture than the health professionals who had negative attitude in their whole life.

Health professionals who had positive attitude were 3.2 times more likely to refer to herbal medicine than those who had negative attitude in their whole life. Nurses were 2.9 and pharmacists 1.3 times more likely to refer to postnatal care than doctors. Health professionals who had positive attitude towards postnatal care were 2.2 times more likely to refer to postnatal care than those who had negative attitude in their whole life.

However, pharmacists were 2.6 times more likely to refer to other types of T&CM than doctors, while nurses were less likely (AOR=0.861) to refer to other types of T&CM. Health professionals who had positive attitude were 4.6 times more likely to refer to other types of T&CM than those who had negative attitude towards T&CM.

Table 4.52 Multivariate logistic regression to determine modalities of T&CM associated with referral of T&CM in the whole life among the health professionals

PRACTICE OF TRADITIONAL AND COMPLEMENTARY MEDICINE AMONG HEALTH PROFESSIONALS IN MALAYSIA

Independent Variable		AOR	95% CI	X^2 df	p-value@
Massage					
Age (year)	<40	1			
	≥40	1.706	1.146-2.54	6.923(1)	0.009**
Religion	Islam	1.595	1.042-2.442	4.616(1)	0.032*
	Non Islam	1			
Attitude	Negative	1			
	Positive	1.659	1.077-2.556	5.272(1)	0.022*
Acupuncture					
Hospital				9.148(4)	0.058
	UKMMC	1			
	HPJ	4.855	1.609-14.652	7.859 (1)	0.005**
	HSNZ	3.639	1.151-11.505	4.838(1)	0.028*
	HDOK	4.075	1.323-12.549	5.993(1)	0.014*
	SGH	2.475	0.779 -7.859	2.362(1)	0.124
				6.193(3)	0.029*
Age	<40	1			
	≥40	1.977	1.071-3.647	4.755(1)	0.029*
				10.083(2)	0.006**
Career	Doctor	1			
	Pharmacist	0.329	0.145-0.746	7.089 (1)	0.008**
	Nurses	0.353	0.158-0.787	6.477 (1)	0.011*
Marital Status	Married	0.468	0.231-0.948	4.448(1)	0.035*
	Not married	1			
Income (RM)	Low (>4000)	1			
	High (≤4000)	2.651	1.298-5.416	7.156(1)	0.007**

Knowledge	Poor	1			
	Good	1.869	1.01-3.458	3.968(1)	0.046*
Attitude	Negative	1			
	Positive	1.98	0.97-4.043	3.52(1)	0.061
Herbal medicine					
Attitude				2.601(2)	0.272
	Negative	1			
	Positive	3.224	1.409-7.38	7.679(1)	0.006**
Postnatal care					
Career				10.376(2)	0.006**
	Doctor	1			
	Pharmacist	1.341	0.552-3.359	0.419(1)	0.517
	Nurse	2.917	1.43-5.949	8.667(1)	0.003**
Attitude	Negative	1			
	Positive	2.236	1.097-4.557	4.907(1)	0.027*
Other types of T&CM					
Career				6.688(2)	0.035
	Doctor	1			
	Pharmacist	2.56	0.952-6.881	3.47(1)	0.062
	Nurse	0.861	0.279-2.661	0.067(1)	0.795
Attitude	Negative	1			
	Positive	4.574	1.339-15.619	5.886(1)	0.015*

Adj. OR = Adjusted odds ratio; [a] Likelihood Ratio (LR) test; [b] Wald test
*significant at p<0.05, **significant at p<0.01, ***significant at p<0.001

Table 4.53 describes the final logistic regression model for referral massage in the last one year with other determinant variables. It shows that health professionals who had positive attitude were 2.3 times more likely to refer to massage therapies than those who had negative attitude.

HDOK was 5.9 times, SGH was 3.8 times, HPJ was 3.6 times and HSNZ was 3.4 times more likely to refer to acupuncture than UKMMC. Doctors were 3.6 times more likely to refer to T&CM than pharmacists and 4.8 times more likely than nurses. High income health professionals were 3.1 times more likely to refer to acupuncture than low income health professionals. The health professionals who had positive attitude were 2.9 times more likely to refer to acupuncture than who had negative attitude towards T&CM in the last one year.

The health professionals who had Bachelor's degree were 3.7 times and Master's or PhD 3.6 times more likely to refer to herbal medicine than who those had diploma. The health professionals who had positive attitude were 6.7 times more likely to refer to herbal medicine than those who had negative attitude towards T&CM in the last one year.

Married health professionals were 3.4 times more likely to refer to postnatal care than the non-married health professionals in the last one year. The health professionals who had positive attitude were 3.3 times more likely refer to other types of T&CM than those who had negative attitude towards T&CM in the last one year.

Table 4.53 Multivariate logistic regression to determine modalities of T&CM associated with referral of T&CM in the last one year among the health professionals

Independent Variable		AOR	95% CI	X^2 df	p-value
Massage					
Attitude	Negative	1			
	Positive	2.309	1.286-4.149	7.842(1)	0.005**
Acupuncture					
Hospital				6.685 (4)	0.153
	UKMMC	1			
	HPJ	3.604	0.901-14.42	3.283 (1)	0.070
	HSNZ	3.369	0.817-13.896	2.822(1)	0.093
	HDOK	5.89	1.518 -22.86	6.569(1)	0.010*
	SGH	3.853	0.967-15.35	3.658(1)	0.056
Career				12.678 (2)	0.002**
	Doctor	1			
	Pharmacist	0.281	0.11-0.717	7.048(1)	0.008**
	Nurse	0.208	0.077-0.564	9.512(1)	0.002**
Income (RM)	Low (>4000)	1			
	High (≤4000)	3.099	1.331-7.215	6.881(1)	0.009**
Attitude	Negative	1			
	Positive	2.873	1.261-6.546	6.31(1)	0.012
Herbal Medicine					
				4.317 (2)	0.116
Education	Diploma	1			
	Degree	3.738	1.047-13.345	4.122(1)	0.042*
	Master/PhD	3.634	0.879-15.017	3.177(1)	0.075
Attitude	Negative	1			
	Positive	6.728	1.548-29.236	6.468(1)	0.011*

Postnatal Care					
Marital Status	Married	3.434	0.997-11.833	3.822(1)	0.051
	Not married	1			
Other types of T&CM treatment					
Attitude	Negative	1			
	Positive	3.26	0.721-14.743	2.356(1)	0.125

Adj. OR = Adjusted odds ratio; [a] Likelihood Ratio (LR) test; [b] Wald test
*significant at p<0.05, **significant at p<0.01

Table 4.54 describes the final logistic regression model for knowledge, attitude towards T&CM and perception in education about T&CM with other determinant variables. It shows that HDOK was 3.2 times, HPJ 2.8 times, HSNZ 1.7 and SGH 1.2 times more likely to have good knowledge of T&CM than UKMMC. Pharmacists were 2.0 times and nurses 1.1 times more knowledgeable in T&CM than doctors, whilst married health professionals had 1.883 times better knowledge than the non-married health professionals.

HSNZ was 3.0 times, HDOK 2.9, HPJ 2.2 and SGH 2.1 times more likely to have positive attitude than UKMMC. The health professionals aged 40 and above were 1.6 times more likely to have more positive attitude than those below 40. Malays have 2.0 times more positive attitude than the non-Malays, while nurses have 3.1 times and pharmacists 2.9 times more positive attitude than doctors towards T&CM.

Female health professionals were 2.1 times more likely to have more positive perception on health education in T&CM than males. Malays have 3.8 times more positive perception on education in T&CM than the non-Malays. Muslim health professionals have 6.1 times more positive perception on education in T&CM than the non-Muslims. Pharmacists have 4.4 times and nurses 1.4 times more positive perception regarding education in T&CM than doctors.

Table 4.54 Multivariable logistic regression to determine knowledge, attitude, and perception on education in T&CM associated with the use of T&CM among the health professionals

Independent Variable		AOR	95% CI	X^2 df	p-value@
Knowledge					
Hospital name				19.773(4)	0.001**
	UKMMC	1			
	HPJ	2.814	1.49-5.31	10.163(1)	0.001
	HSNZ	1.726	0.90-3.303	2.723(1)	0.990
	HDOK	3.16	1.64-6.089	11.828(1)	0.001**
	SGH	1.25	0.63-2.455	0.42(1)	0.517
Career				8.136(2)	0.017*
	Doctors	1			
	Pharmacists	1.992	1.217-3.26	7.522(1)	0.006**
	Nurses	1.132	0.707-1.81	0.267(1)	0.605
Marital	Married	1.883	1.204-2.94	7.699(1)	0.006**
	Not married	1			

PRACTICE OF TRADITIONAL AND COMPLEMENTARY MEDICINE AMONG HEALTH PROFESSIONALS IN MALAYSIA

Attitude					
Hospital Name				15.67(4)	0.003**
	UKMMC	1			
	HPJ	2.251	1.197-4.23	6.338(1)	0.012*
	HSNZ	3.012	1.551-5.84	10.598(1)	0.001**
	HDOK	2.905	1.521-5.54	10.426(1)	0.001**
	SGH	2.127	1.115-4.06	5.243(1)	0.022*
Age (year)	<40	1			
	≥40	1.626	1.044-2.53	4.633	0.031*
Ethnicity	Malays	1.98	1.21-3.24	7.398(1)	0.007**
	Non-Malays	1			
Career				26.652(2)	<0.001***
	Doctor	1			
	Pharmacist	2.902	1.721-4.89	15.959(1)	<0.001***
	Nurse	3.143	1.93-5.102	21.451(1)	<0.001***
Perception					
Sex	Male	1			
	Female	2.07	1.124-3.81	5.446(1)	0.020*

Adj. OR = Adjusted odds ratio; [a] Likelihood Ratio (LR) test; [b] Wald test
*significant at p<0.05, **significant at p<0.01, ***significant at p<0.001

DR. MAGFIRET A. BOZLAR, PROF. DR. SYED ALJUNID

QUALITATIVE STUDY ON PRACTICE OF T&CM

Introduction

Part B of the questionnaire was used as a basis to conduct this qualitative study. The study was designed to assess the opinion of the health professionals in five selected hospitals in Malaysia on their perception of their practice of T&CM in Malaysia, usage and recommendation of T&CM, knowledge on T&CM, integrating T&CM into Western Medicine, and opinion on future medical training in T&CM respectively. A total of ten health professionals were chosen from the five hospitals in the qualitative study. Equal numbers of Malays and non-Malays as well as Muslims and non-Muslims were involved in this study.

Ten health professionals had given their consent to participate in the qualitative study. The youngest participant was 26 years old and the oldest 58. Eight of the participants were married and two were single. One of the participants was a professor who had a PhD degree. Most of the health professionals interviewed had a bachelor degree.

4.54 Socio-demographic characteristics of the participants (n=10)

Variables	Number of Participants	Percentage (%)
Hospitals		
UKMMC	2	20.0

HPJ	2	20.0
HSNZ	2	20.0
HDOK	2	20.0
SGH	2	20.0
Age		
<40	5	50.0
≥40	5	50.0
Gender		
Male	4	40.0
Female	6	60.0
Ethnicity		
Malay	5	50.0
Non-Malay	5	50.0
Religion		
Islam	5	50.0
Non-Islam	5	50.0
Career		
Doctors	3	30.0
Pharmacist	4	40.0
Nurses	3	30.0
Years of Working		
≤10	4	40.0
>10	6	60.0
Marital Status		
Married	8	80.0
Unmarried	2	20.0

Education Level		
Diploma	1	10.0
Degree	6	60.0
Master/PhD	3	30.0
Income (RM)		
Low (<4000)	4	40.0
High (≥4000)	6	60.0

An in-depth interview was carried out which consisted of seven domains that described the practice of T&CM among health professionals in Malaysia namely (1) Opinion on popularity of using T&CM among the population (2) Opinion on reasons for using T&CM (3) Practice of T&CM (4) Prescribing or recommending T&CM, T&CM practitioners and reasons for recommending it (5) Knowledge of T&CM (6) Do you think that T&CM can be integrated with WM? Please explain (7) Opinion on T&CM being a part of future training for medical students.

Opinion on Popularity of Using T&CM among the Population

Most participants (9) agreed with the statement that Traditional and Complementary Medicine is popular among the population in Malaysia. One respondent does not want his patients to use T&CM although he agreed that T&CM is popular.

"It is very popular among the population." **(Malay, 52, pharmacist, married, master's degree)**

"It is quite popular especially among the rural population as well as in Sandakan." **(Indian, 34, doctor, married, master's degree)**

"I think T&CM is quite popular. Generally, people would use T&CM when WM fails. Some people in Sarawak before trying WM would prefer to use T&CM. I think they do not take tablets or capsules but use a natural way of taking whole herbs. Sometimes they cook whole herbs" **(Chinese, 30, pharmacist, married, bachelor's degree)**

"It is popular among the population. But I am against the use of T&CM for patients." **(Malay, 52 years, specialist, married, PhD)**

Opinion on Reasons for Using Traditional and Complementary Medicine

Most participants thought that people trusted in T&CM and were afraid of WM.

"People don't need to see the doctor. People consider that there is no side effect. They don't know the side effect of T&CM until they get sick." **(Malay, 52 years, pharmacist, married, master's degree)**

*"Many people are scared of using WM. They believe that WM is harmful to the health and has many side effects. I support the use of T&CM in combination with WM. I think traditional

medicine is useful for minor illnesses." **(Chinese, male, 29, pharmacist, unmarried, bachelor's degree)**

"People believe that T&CM is good for chronic diseases. Sometimes WM doesn't work. In Terengganu many people believed in Islamic medicine as well." **(Malay, female, 58, nurse, married, diploma)**

"People believed in T&CM. Sometimes when western medicine does not work, people seek help from T&CM. Maybe it is the last choice by using T&CM. Actually many people believed in T&CM and it is effective because it works." **(Malay, female, 32, pharmacist, married, bachelor's degree)**

"Effect would be better than taking just WM. A lot of people are concerned with side effect of WM. People think that natural things are safer." **(Chinese, female, 37, pharmacist, married, bachelor's degree)**

Some participants believed that T&CM is easily available and cheaper than WM.

"Easy access. It is easily available. People don't need to see the doctor. It is cheap." **(Malay, 52, pharmacist, married, master's degree)**

"It is widely and easily available. It is also cheaper than WM. No need to see the doctors." **(Chinese, female, 26, pharmacist, unmarried, bachelor's degree)**

"It is easily available. People are afraid to go to the Western Medical Hospital especially when some procedures need to

be done such as CT-scan, blood test, etc." *(Malay, male, 53, doctor, married, PhD)*

Practice of Traditional and Complementary Medicine

All the participants used some types of Traditional and Complementary Medicine personally.

"I am using herbs for myself to control my blood sugar and high blood pressure. I am using 'misai kucing' and it is very good." *(Malay, male, 55, doctor, married, bachelor's degree)*

"One day when I woke up I could not move my neck. After using a few needles I felt the pain was gone very quickly. I had undergone Chinese massage after acupuncture. From that time, whenever I have back pain or neck pain or very bad posture I go for acupuncture." *(Chinese, male, 29, pharmacist unmarried, bachelor's degree)*

"I used T&CM such as acupuncture, traditional massage, postnatal care, herbal medicine, homeopathy and Islamic medicine. I used acupuncture when I had very terrible pain and I could not open my mouth. After using acupuncture, I saw a good result, then I automatically continue using it." *(Malay, female, 58, nurse, married, diploma)*

"I used T&CM especially for postnatal care. I believe in T&CM. I have used massage and herbal medicine for my back pain and headache. Even T&CM is good for fracture of bone. My sister had two fractures in her bones. The shape of her arms was very bad. My parents brought her to a 'bomoh' for treatment. After

2-3 months later her hand recovered. She now can carry heavy things like a normal person." *(Malay, female, 32, pharmacist, married, bachelor's degree)*

Prescribing or Recommending T&CM, T&CM Practitioners and Reason for Recommending it

Most of the respondents generally recommended T&CM for treatment, but since pharmacists and nurses do not have the rights to prescribe, they have not prescribed T&CM to their patients.

"I recommend certain T&CM products such as ginger, garlic pills and lemongrass because I know of their health benefits. I know that lemongrass and some other herbs are good for toothache so I recommend them to others." *(Malay, male, 55, doctor, married, bachelor's degree)*

"Since I am a pharmacist I have not recommended it to the patients but I recommend acupuncture to my friends. I am really aware of herbal medicine's side effect. I have recommended T&CM to my friends when' they did not get well from their illnesses after using WM for a long time." *(Chinese, female, 26, pharmacist, unmarried, bachelor's degree)*

"I recommended acupuncture to my father when he got neck pain, and a traditional Malay massage to my mother when she had lower back pain. I have recommended traditional treatment to my patients and colleagues for lower back pain because of my experience and belief." *(Chinese, male, 29, Pharmacist unmarried, bachelor's degree)*

PRACTICE OF TRADITIONAL AND COMPLEMENTARY MEDICINE AMONG HEALTH PROFESSIONALS IN MALAYSIA

"I cannot prescribe T&CM but I have advised some patients to use T&CM through a doctor. Many post-stroke patients got good result from adopting T&CM. It depends on the patients' health condition." **(Bidayuh, female, 40, nurse, married, diploma)**

Half of the health professionals referred their patients or family members to T&CM practitioners, but some of them did not even know where and whom to refer to.

"I refer patients to T&CM doctors for massage, postnatal care and Islamic medicine as well, but not herbal treatments. Because I know them better than herbal medicine and others." **(Malay, 52, pharmacist, married, master's degree)**

"I personally don't know of any qualified T&CM practitioner." **(Chinese, female, 26, pharmacist, unmarried, bachelor's degree)**

"We don't have contacts with T&CM doctors. So, I cannot refer cases to T&CM doctors. Actually, patients have asked us to refer them to T&CM and some of my patients have also asked me to recommend T&CM for them. T&CM people here did not publicize their service. That is why many doctors do not refer to them". **(Indian, male, 34, doctor, married, master's degree)**

"I do not know where the T&CM practitioners are available. I think there is no T&CM doctor. I think patients should go for both, not only WM but also T&CM. I read many cases of cancer patients going to T&CM doctors for T&CM treatments only but the treatments only delayed the progression of their diseases." **(Chinese, male, 29, unmarried, bachelor's degree)**

DR. MAGFIRET A. BOZLAR, PROF. DR. SYED ALJUNID

Knowledge of Traditional and Complementary Medicine

All the health professionals believed that T&CM has therapeutic value. Most of them believed so because of their personal experience. Some of them believed in it because they have read some articles about it.

"I believed that T&CM has therapeutic value. I can say that from my own practice. I am a doctor and I have a colleague who is also a doctor but I do not ask him to use herbal medicine. It is difficult for me to convince the doctor about the use of herbs." **(Malay, male, 55, doctor, married, bachelor's degree)**

"I personally believed that T&CM has therapeutic value because I have tried some herbs and seen good results. I also believed that if there is no therapeutic value, why people have used it for so long since thousands and hundreds of years ago until now. If there were no therapeutic value in them, by now it would have been extinct." **(Chinese, female, 26, pharmacist, unmarried, bachelor's degree)**

"Actually I have been suffering from trigeminalgia nervosa on the left side of my face since 2004. I went to every clinic to find a cure. My pain recurred for 2 years. A doctor gave me WM and also advised me to use T&CM. I used only acupuncture for more than 20 cycles already. I really have seen good result. The pain was relieved after using acupuncture. There was no more acute pain as before." **(Malay, female, 58, nurse, married, diploma)**

"I believed T&CM has therapeutic value. I have read a lot of articles and watched TV channels about T&CM. I have interviewed a patient who had numbness and used painkiller but it didn't work. Finally, she used a T&CM treatment then she had very good result. She now works like normal people." **(Malay, female, 32, pharmacist, married, bachelor's degree)**

Opinion of Integration of T&CM into Western Medicine

Everybody agreed with a statement on an integration of T&CM with WM except two respondents who worked in a non-integrated hospital (UKMMC). Because they considered UKMMC as a teaching hospital, it should not be integrated unless it was an evidence-based modality. But they accepted to having a T&CM unit in other hospitals.

"Why not? T&CM has been developed from experience that led to a certain conclusion on its effectiveness. The only advantage of WM is that it has properly and systematically been proven through real evidence. There are thousands of people who refuse conventional medicine seem to have benefited from T&CM. It means there is evidence." **(Indian, male, 34, doctor, married, master's degree)**

"I think T&CM can be integrated with WM. I think T&CM has additional benefits and synergistic effect for some medical conditions." **(Chinese, female, 37, pharmacist, married, bachelor's degree)**

"Yes, according to my experience. We have to combine WM and T&CM. because WM gives immediate effects. T&CM effects

are slow but the result lasts a long time. Both of them have their own benefits. Nowadays, many doctors in Terengganu advise their patients to use T&CM. The Ministry of Health has to set up a T&CM unit in every hospital in Malaysia." **(Malay, female, 58, nurse, married, diploma)**

"I think T&CM can be integrated with WM. Some T&CM treatments have evidence. So, whichever that has evidence should be integrated with WM. If it is evidence-based, it can be integrated with WM even in a teaching hospital. There should be a T&CM unit or T&CM practitioners in WM hospitals." **(Malay, female, 52, pharmacist, married, master's degree)**

Opinion on T&CM being a Part of Future Training for Medical Students

Most respondents agreed for T&CM to be a part of future training for health professionals. However, some of them wanted it to be optional for the students. Only one respondent did not agree with this statement.

"I think it would be good if T&CM can be part of future training for medical students because they should have an exposure to T&CM and know about T&CM." **(Malay, female, 32, pharmacist, married, bachelor's degree)**

"I think T&CM should be part of future training for medical students as well as health professionals. I also want to learn about T&CM that relates to acupuncture, massaging and herbal medicine if I have the opportunity." **(Bidayuh, female, 40, nurse, married, diploma)**

PRACTICE OF TRADITIONAL AND COMPLEMENTARY MEDICINE AMONG HEALTH PROFESSIONALS IN MALAYSIA

"They should be given a freedom to choose whether or not they want to learn T&CM. I don't think everyone trust T&CM especially among the medical students because for them the whole idea is to become a doctor in a Western Medical hospital." **(Chinese, female, 26, pharmacist, unmarried, bachelor's degree)**

SUMMARY

A total of ten health professionals were enrolled from selected five hospitals. Two health professionals from each hospital participated in this qualitative study. A total of six females and four males were interviewed for the study. Five of the health professionals were at the age of 40 years or older while the remaining five were younger than 40. Most of them believed that T&CM was popular among health professionals in Malaysia.

The survey of opinion on the reasons for using T&CM suggested that most of the health professionals believed that "people use T&CM because they are afraid of side effects of WM and also their easy access.

From the interview, it shows that all the participants have experienced in using some types of T&CM in their life for whatever reason they might have. About half of the health professionals have recommended T&CM to their patients or family members in their life. However, a small number of health professionals have negative idea about T&CM but all the health professionals interviewed believed that some types of T&CM have therapeutic value.

Apparently everybody agreed on an integration of T&CM with WM, while some of the health professionals believed that T&CM should be part of future medical training. However, some of them wanted to give a freedom of choice to health professionals whether they want it or not. There was only one health professionals who disagreed on the integration of the two disciplines but yet he agreed for T&CM to be a part of future training for pharmacy students only.

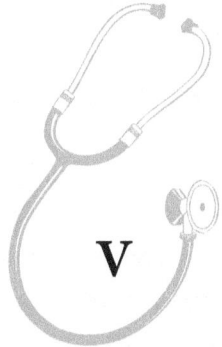

V

DISCUSSION

This section reports the discussion about the practice of T&CM among health professionals and factors related to it among health professionals in five selected hospitals in Malaysia namely UKMMC, HPJ, HSNZ, HDOK and SGH. In this cross-sectional study the use of T&CM during whole life, the use of T&CM in the last one year, T&CM referral during whole life and T&CM referral in the last one year were recorded among the health professionals. Socio-demographic characteristics of health professionals, modalities of T&CM use, knowledge regarding T&CM, attitude towards T&CM and perception on education about T&CM and reason of using and not using T&CM were measured and analyzed by using univariate analysis, bivariate analysis and multivariable analysis.

DR. MAGFIRET A. BOZLAR, PROF. DR. SYED ALJUNID

THE RATE OF T&CM USE AND REFERRAL

Use of T&CM during Whole Life and in the Last One Year

The study investigated the use of T&CM, T&CM referral during whole life, use of T&CM and T&CM referral in the last one year among health professionals. The study results revealed some general trends. Almost half of the health professionals (46.3%) used T&CM during whole life, and also almost the same amount of health professionals (48.6%) referred T&CM to patients and their family members during whole life.

Approximately one in third of the health professionals (32.5%) used T&CM in the last one year while a quarter of health professionals (25.2%) referred T&CM to patients and their family members in the last one year. A total of two thirds of the health professionals (67.5%) had ever personally practiced (used or recommended) T&CM to their patients and family in their life and almost half of them (45.9%) used or recommended T&CM to patients and family members in the last one year. It indicates that most of the health professionals used or recommended T&CM to their patients or family.

MODALITIES OF T&CM

There are some differences in the use/referral of massage, acupuncture, herbal medicine, postnatal care and other types of T&CM among the health professionals during whole life and in the last one year. Bivariate and multivariable analysis provided the clear picture about modalities of T&CM.

Approximately 20% of the health professionals have used massage (21.4%), herbal therapies (19.5%) and postnatal care (18.7%) during their lifetime. However, fewer participants used T&CM in the last one year, in which the use of massage (13.0%) was the highest in comparison to others. In contrast, Xu and Levine (2008) stressed that thirty-eight percent of the medical residents had never personally used herbal medicine but in this study 84.3% doctors had never personally used herbal medicine in their life. This is probably because herbal medicine is not really accepted by the doctors in Malaysia as compared to the doctors in China.

More than 30.0% of health professionals referred to massage and around 13.0% referred to acupuncture and postnatal care in their whole life. This is probably because a total of 85.1% health professionals believed that massage could help in maintaining physical, mental, and emotional well-being. As much as twice the number of respondents (16.4%) referred to massage than acupuncture (8.6%) in the last one year but in another study (Massimo et al. 2007), more than two-thirds (69.2%) of general practitioners (GPs) recommended acupuncture in Italy. Only 6.6% doctors referred T&CM in this study. In contrast, 80% of physicians prescribed phytomedicines in Germany (Thomas et al. 2008). This is probably because herbal medicine service has not been started in Malaysian hospitals yet and also due to lack of knowledge about T&CM among health professionals in Malaysia.

The findings of the study showed that there was no significant association between use and referral of herbal medicine and socio-demographic characteristics of the respondents during their whole life and in the last one year. Herbal medicine is integrated with western medicine in some western medical hospitals such as Hospital Sultan Ismail and Hospital Kepala Batas, still however, it is not integrated into these selected hospitals yet.

The use of different types of T&CM modalities such as massage, acupuncture, herbal medicine, postnatal care and others types of T&CM was not high compared to other study, however the use of massage, herbal medicine and postnatal care is higher than acupuncture and other types of herbal medicine.

Massage and acupuncture referral were not high as compared to other study, however their referral were also higher as compared to other types of T&CM modalities. It shows that health professionals accepted massage and acupuncture. Since integration of herbal medicine has not yet taken place at the hospitals' T&CM unit yet, use of herbal medicine and herbal medicine referral were still low.

ASSOCIATION BETWEEN USE/REFERRAL OF T&CM AND SOCIO-DEMOGRAPHIC CHARACTERISTICS OF HEALTH PROFESSIONALS

The study investigates the association between use/referral of T&CM and socio-demographic characteristics of health

PRACTICE OF TRADITIONAL AND COMPLEMENTARY MEDICINE AMONG HEALTH PROFESSIONALS IN MALAYSIA

professionals by using bivariate analysis and multivariable analysis. The finding shows that there was a relationship between use/referral of T&CM and socio-demographic characteristics of the health professionals.

Use/Referral of T&CM among the Hospitals

The study compared the use/referral of T&CM among five selected hospitals by using bivariate analysis and multivariable analysis. The findings indicate that among five selected hospitals, the use of massage was significantly higher among the health professionals in HDOK. Almost one-third of the health professionals (31.6%) in HDOK used massage (p=0.045). Health professionals of HDOK were 1.7 times more likely to use massage therapy as compared to that of UKMMC. However, UKMMC health professionals were 1.37, 1.46 and 1.7 times more likely to use massage as compared to health professionals in HPJ, HSNZ and SGH during their whole life. Although UKMMC is not the T&CM integrated hospital, the use of massage was higher than the three T&CM integrated hospitals (p=0.018).

As far as the use of postnatal care is concerned, the finding of this study showed that almost half of the health professionals (46.3%) used postnatal care in Hospital Putrajaya (p=0.03). The health professionals at Hospital Duchess of Kent (HDOK) were almost 4 times (3.975 times), Hospital Putrajaya (HPJ) were more than 3.5 times (3.619 times) (p=0.004), Sarawak General Hospital (SGH) and Hospital Sultanah Nur Zahirah (HSNZ) were more than 2.5 times (2.709 and 2.676 times respectively) more likely to use postnatal care than those at UKMMC in their whole life. Postnatal care services are available in four T&CM integrated hospitals except UKMMC.

Regarding acupuncture, the finding shows that acupuncture referral was significantly higher at HPJ (20%, p=0.026) and HPJ was approximately five times (4.855 times) (p=0.005), HDOK four times (4.075 times) (p=0.014), HSNZ more than 3.5 times (3.639 times) (p=0.028) and SGH almost 2.5 times (2.475 times) more likely to refer patients/family to acupuncture than UKMMC in their whole life. Moreover, HDOK was almost six times (5.89 times) (p=0.01), SGH was almost four times (3.853), HPJ was almost 3.5 times (3.604 times) and HSNZ was about 3.5 times (3.369 times) more likely to refer patients/family to acupuncture than UKMMC in the last one year. Since the other four hospitals are T&CM-integrated hospitals, acupuncture is available at these four hospitals but there is no service of acupuncture at UKMMC since it is not the T&CM-integrated hospital.

Meanwhile, HSNZ was almost 4.5 times (4.463) and SGH was about 2.5 times (2.772 times) more likely to use other types of T&CM than UKMMC. However, UKMMC was 1.3 times and 1.75 times more likely to use other types of T&CM than HDOK and HPJ respectively in the last one year.

The use of massage was highest among health professionals in HDOK as compared to other hospitals. However, although UKMMC is not the T&CM-integrated hospital, the use of massage was higher in which it falls second after HDOK. The use of postnatal care was higher among married female health professionals in HDOK and HPJ than others. Acupuncture referral was higher in HPJ and HDOK as compared to others. The use of other types of T&CM was higher in HSNZ, mainly because the hospital used Islamic medicine. The main population in Kuala Terengganu is Muslim and Kuala Terengganu is considered as the Islamic state in Malaysia.

Association between Use/Referral of T&CM and Age

Regarding age, this study showed that more than half of the health professionals aged 40 years and older (55.7%) were more likely to refer patients or their family members to T&CM in their whole life (p=0.014). Less than half of the health professionals aged 40 years and older (41.0%) more likely to refer massage to their patients and family in their whole life (p=0.002). The health professionals who had more than 10 years of working experience were 1.7 times more likely to refer T&CM to their patients/family as compared to health professionals who had less than 10 years of service in their whole life (p=0.009).

Acupuncture referral is high among health professionals aged 40 years and older (19.7%, p=0.002). The health professionals aged 40 years and older were almost two times more likely to refer acupuncture than health professionals whose age were below 40 years old (p=0.029) during their whole life. In contrast, health professionals at the age below 40 were almost 2.4 times more likely to use other types of T&CM in their whole life (p=0.005).

Overall, T&CM referral, massage and acupuncture were higher among the senior health professionals than their younger colleagues. However, the use of other types of T&CM

was higher among the health professionals that are at the age below 40 as compared to the older staff. There was no significant relationship between use of postnatal care and postnatal care referral during whole life and in the last one year with age.

Association between Use/Referral of T&CM and Gender

Approximately half of the female health professionals (49.9%) used T&CM while one third of male health professionals (34.3%) used T&CM in their whole life (p=0.004). Female respondents were 1.5 times more likely to use T&CM compared to male respondents in their whole life. However, finding showed that more than one-third (36.0%) of female respondents used T&CM (p=0.002). Female health professionals were nearly two times (1.885 times) more likely to use T&CM compared to male health professionals (p=0.018) in one year. Interestingly, more than one-third (36.1%) of male health professionals referred T&CM to their patients and family (p=0.003) and multivariable regression revealed that male health professionals were 2.3 times more likely to refer T&CM to patients/family than female health professionals (p=0.001) in the last one year.

Male health professionals (9.3%) were more likely to use other types of T&CM (p=0.022) as compared to female health professionals during whole life. Male health professionals were 2.5 times and 3.8 times more likely to use other types of T&CM in their whole life (p=0.032) and in the last one year (p=0.017), respectively.

There is no significant association between the use of acupuncture in the whole life and gender. However, the finding shows that referral of acupuncture was significantly higher among male health professionals (20.4%, p=0.02) in the whole life and (14.8%, p=0.009) in the last one year. However, there was no significant association between the use of acupuncture and gender either in the whole life or in the last one year among the health professionals. Female health professionals (15.7%) were more likely to refer postnatal care than male health professionals (p=0.003) in their whole life.

Although the use of T&CM was higher among the female health professionals, T&CM referral was higher among the male health professionals. The use of other types of T&CM was higher among the male health professionals. Referral of acupuncture was significantly higher among male health professionals while postnatal care referral was higher among female health professionals. The personal experience of female health professionals might influence them to refer postnatal care to their patients/family members.

Association between Use/Referral of T&CM and Ethnicity

The study also investigates the association between use/referral of T&CM and ethnicity. The finding shows that there was an association between use/referral of T&CM and ethnicity in which more than one third of Malay health professionals used T&CM in the last one year (p= 0.048). The non-Malays were more likely to use acupuncture than Malay health professionals in their whole life and in the last one year (p=0.002 and p=0.010, respectively).

Malay married female health professionals were more likely to use postnatal care in their whole life and in the last one year. More than one-third of them (38.9%) and 20% of them used postnatal care in their whole life and in the last one year (p=0.032 and p=0.001 respectively). Malay health professionals were 2.3 times and almost 6 times more likely to practice postnatal care than non-Malay health professionals in their whole life and in the last one year (p=0.034, p=0.002 respectively). Twice as much as Malay health professionals (16.6%) were more likely to refer postnatal care than non-Malays (8.5%) (p=0.01) in their whole life.

More than one-third of Malay health professionals (36.5%) referred massage (p=0.029) in their whole life. There was no significant association between referral of massage, acupuncture, herbal medicine, postnatal care and other types of T&CM and ethnicity in their whole life and in the last one year among the health professionals.

Overall, T&CM use, use of postnatal care and massage referral were higher among the Malay health professionals than the non-Malay health professionals. However, use of acupuncture was higher among the non-Malay health professionals.

Association between Use/Referral of T&CM and Religion

The study also investigates the association between use/referral of T&CM and religion. More than one-third of

PRACTICE OF TRADITIONAL AND COMPLEMENTARY MEDICINE AMONG HEALTH PROFESSIONALS IN MALAYSIA

Muslim health professionals (36.1%) used T&CM in the last one year than non-Muslims (26.3%) (p=0.028). As many as half of Muslim health professionals (53%) referred T&CM to their patients and family in their whole life (p= 0.013). Muslim health professionals were 1.4 times more likely to refer T&CM in their whole life than non-Muslim health professionals.

Meanwhile, non-Muslim health professionals were more likely to use acupuncture than Muslim health professionals in their whole life and in the last one year (p=0.001 and p=0.002, respectively). The finding shows that non-Muslims were 4.7 times and 5 times more likely to use acupuncture than Muslim health professionals in their whole life and in the last one year (p=0.004 and 0.017, respectively).

As many as twice married female Muslim health professionals (16.2%) used postnatal care than non-Muslims (8%) in their whole life (p=0.011). Muslim health professionals were more likely to use postnatal care (19.1%) than non-Muslims in the last one year (p=0.003).

More than one-third of (37.1%) Muslim health professionals referred massage to their patients/family in their whole life (p=0.005). Muslim health professionals were 1.6 times more likely to refer massage to their patients/family than non-Muslim health professionals during their whole life (p=0.032).

The use and referral of T&CM were higher among Muslim health professionals. The use of acupuncture however was higher among the non-Muslim health professionals. The use of postnatal care was higher among the Muslim married female health professionals. Massage referral was also higher among the Muslim health professionals.

Association between Use/referral of T&CM and Types of Occupation

This study investigates the association between use/referral of T&CM and type of occupation health professionals; namely doctors, pharmacists and nurses.

In term of type of occupation, the finding shows that more than half of the nurses used T&CM in their whole life (56.2%) while less than half of pharmacists (43.0%) and more than one-third of doctors (39.2%) used it (p=0.005).

About 39.2% doctors have ever used T&CM in their whole life. The finding supports the study by Sikand (1998) who found that 37% of medical doctors used any CAM in their personal lives. In another study by Fountain-Polley (2007), 30% of doctors had personally used CAMs.

A study by Massimo et al. (2007) reported that more than half of the general practitioners (GPs) (58.0%) recommended CAM but only 13.0% used it. In this study, almost the same proportion of health professionals used and recommended T&CM to their patients and family.

Among the general practitioners in Doha, Qatar, it was found that 30.1% had used CAM (Al Shaar et al. 2010). Another study has shown that use of T&CM by doctors was 39.2%; This supported the statement that use of CAM by primary care physicians vary greatly across countries, ranging from

PRACTICE OF TRADITIONAL AND
COMPLEMENTARY MEDICINE AMONG HEALTH
PROFESSIONALS IN MALAYSIA

20.0% and 38.0% in Australia, 30% in New Zealand, 47% in the Netherlands, and up to 95% in Germany (Giannelli et al. 2007).

Doctors were three times more likely to refer acupuncture (23.5%) than pharmacists (8.5%) and nurses (8.3%) to the patients/family in their whole life (p<0.001). Doctors were also three times more likely to refer acupuncture (16.9%) than pharmacists (4.9%) and nurses (3.6%) in the last one year (p<0.001).

The same trend appeared in the multivariable analysis where doctors were three times more likely to refer acupuncture than pharmacists and nurses in their whole life (p=0.006). Doctors were 3.6 times more likely to refer acupuncture than pharmacists and 4.8 times more likely to refer acupuncture than nurses in the last one year (p=0.002). Only 29% of GPs used some types of CAM for themselves. A total of 39.2% GPs used herbs (Ozcadir et al. 2007). Among the Western-trained doctors using TCM, 90.6% used herbal remedies, 32.4% used acupuncture and 5.8% used massage in Shenyang, China in 2001(Harmworth & Lewith 2001).

Pharmacists were more likely to refer other types of T&CM than doctors and nurses in their whole life (p=0.017). Multivariable analysis showed that pharmacists were 2.6 times and doctors were 1.2 times more likely to refer other types of T&CM in their whole life (p=0.035).

Meanwhile, nurses were more likely to use massage in their whole life and in the last one year than pharmacists and doctors. One-third of nurses have experienced massage

(29.0%) in their whole life and 18.9% used it in the last one year (p=0.009 and p=0.011, respectively). Multivariable analysis showed that nurses were 2.4 times and doctors were 1.25 times more likely to use massage than pharmacists in the last one year (p=0.004). Nurses were more likely to refer massage (39.1%) than doctors (34.3%) and pharmacists (22.5%) in their whole life (p=0.007).

Nurses were three times more likely to refer to postnatal care (23.7%) than pharmacists (7.7%) and doctors (7.2%) during their whole life (p<0.001). Almost the same trend appeared in the multivariable analysis, nurses were three times and pharmacists were 1.3 times more likely to refer postnatal care than doctors in their whole life (p=0.006).

A study by Samuels et al. (2010) showed that 87.3% nurse-midwives used CAM in Israel. Our findings is not as high as reported in this study, however, both studies showed many nurses used T&CM. Among all CAM therapies, 67.1%, 48.6%, 42.2%, 40.5% and 39.9% nurse-midwives used massage, herbal medicine, meditation, touch therapies and prayer respectively in Israel.

Among the health professionals, nurses were more likely to use T&CM than pharmacists and doctors in their whole life. Nurses were also more likely to use/refer massage than others. Married female nurses were more likely to refer postnatal care than others. Doctors were more likely to refer acupuncture than pharmacists and nurses. Pharmacists were more likely to refer other types of T&CM than others.

PRACTICE OF TRADITIONAL AND COMPLEMENTARY MEDICINE AMONG HEALTH PROFESSIONALS IN MALAYSIA

Association between Use/Referral of T&CM and Years of Working

This study also investigates the association between use/referral of T&CM and years of working among the health professionals. The comparison was made between health professionals who have 10 years or less working experience and those who have more than 10 years of working experience.

In terms of years of working, half of the health professionals (50.8%) who have more than 10 years of working experience used T&CM while 40.9% health professionals who have 10 years or less working experience used T&CM in their whole life (p= 0.032).

More than half of the health professionals (55.3%) who have more than 10 years of working experience referred T&CM while only 40.5% health professionals who have less than 10 years of working experience referred T&CM to their patients and family during their whole life (p=0.001). Multivariable analysis showed that health professionals who have more than 10 years of working experience were 1.7 times more likely to refer T&CM in their whole life than health professionals who have 10 years or less working experience (p=0.009).

Married female health professionals who have 10 or less years of working experience (21.4%) were almost twice more likely to use postnatal care than married female health professionals who have more than 10 years of working experience (12.1%) in the last one year (p=0.049). Married female health professionals who have 10 years or less working experience were 2.3 times more likely to use postnatal care in the last one year (p=0.025). This is probably because health professionals whith less working experience are younger and more reproductive.

Meanwhile, as many as one-third of health professionals (38.9%) who have more than 10 years of working experience referred massage during their whole life (p=0.001).

Twice as much health professionals (16.8%) who have more than 10 years of working experience as compared to health professionals who have 10 years or less working experience (8.8%) referred postnatal care during their whole life (p=0.011).

However, there was no significant association between the use of other types of T&CM in the last one year and years of working among the health professionals. Health professionals who have more than 10 years of working experience were 4.4 times more likely to use other types of T&CM in the last one year (p=0.026).

In contrast, younger and more recently trained physicians were more likely to recommend CAM as compared to their older and more experienced colleagues. This is probably because of the increased exposure of younger physicians to CAM in the past decade or there is a higher likelihood that younger physicians used CAM themselves (Maidi et al. 2008).

The use/referral of T&CM was higher among the senior health professionals as compared to their younger colleagues. Senior health professionals were more likely to use postnatal care as compared to younger health professionals. This could probably be due to senior health professionals have more children and more exposured to postnatal care as compared to young health professionals. Senior health professionals were more likely to refer postnatal care and massage than younger health professionals.

Association between Use/Referral of T&CM and Marital Status

The study investigates the association between use/referral of T&CM and marital status of the health professionals. Half of the married health professionals (52.3%) used T&CM while fewer unmarried health professionals (35.5%) used T&CM during their whole life (p<0.001). One-third of married health professionals (36.0%) used T&CM while only 26.0% unmarried health professionals used T&CM in the last one year (p=0.026).

Multivariable analysis showed that married health professionals were twice more likely to use T&CM than unmarried health professionals in their whole life (p<0.001) and 1.5 times more likely to use T&CM than unmarried health professionals in the last one year (p=0.072).

A quarter of married health professionals (25.6%) used massage while 13.6% unmarried health professionals used it in their whole life (p=0.002). Married health professionals have use twice as much massage than unmarried health professionals in the last one year (p=0.023). Multivariable analysis revealed that married health professionals were 2.4 times more likely to use massage than unmarried health professionals in their whole life (p=0.001).

Meanwhile, unmarried health professionals were almost four times more likely to use acupuncture than married health professionals in the last one year (p=0.01). This is probably because unmarried health professionals have more physical activities such as exercise and sport that causes them to have body pain easily. The acupuncture is used to relieve the pain.

Multivariable analysis showed that unmarried health professionals were two times and three times more likely to refer acupuncture than married health professionals in their whole life (p=0.035) and in the last one year respectively.

The rate of using other types of T&CM was not high, in which unmarried health professionals were two times more likely to use other types of T&CM as compared to married health professionals in the last one year (p=0.04). The findings revealed that unmarried health professionals were four times more likely to use other types of T&CM than married health professionals in the last one year (p=0.017).

Referral of postnatal care was six times higher among married health professionals than unmarried health professionals in their whole life (p<0.001) and three times higher in the last one year (p=0.038). Married health professionals were 3.4 times more likely to refer postnatal care than unmarried health professionals in the last one year.

The use of T&CM was higher among married health professionals. The use of massage was higher among married health professionals than unmarried health professionals maybe because they were more likely to take care of themselves than unmarried health professionals. Interestingly,

Unmarried health professionals were more likely to use acupuncture than married health professionals. Unmarried health professionals were also more likely to use other types of T&CM than married health professionals. Postnatal care referral was higher among the married health professionals. This is probably because they also have experience in using postnatal care.

Association between Use/Referral of T&CM and Education Level

The study investigates the association between use/referral of T&CM and education level. As far as education level is concerned, statistical analysis indicated that there was no relationship between use/referral of T&CM and education level.

Association between Use/Referral of T&CM and Income

The study also investigates the association between use/referral of T&CM and income; Income of the health professionals was categorized into low income health professionals (RM<4000) and high income health professionals (RM≥4000).

Multivariable analysis revealed that high income health professionals (20.1%) were more likely to refer acupuncture than low income health professionals (7.9%) in their whole life (p<0.001). Moreover, high income health professionals were four times more likely to refer acupuncture than low income health professionals (p<0.001).

The study also revealed that low income health professionals were 1.5 times more likely to use T&CM as compared to the high-income health professionals in their whole life (p=0.041). However, high income health professionals were 1.5 times more likely to refer T&CM to their patients/family in the last one year.

Statistical analysis showed that high income health professionals were 1.7 times more likely to use massage and three times more likely to refer massage than low income health professionals in the last one year (p= 0.009).

In conclusion, low income health professionals were more likely to use T&CM; high income health professionals were more likely to refer T&CM as compared to low income health professionals in their whole life. Acupuncture referral was higher among the high income health professionals. The use of massage and massage referral were higher among high income health professionals as compared to low-income health professionals in the last one year.

ASSOCIATION BETWEEN THE USE OF T&CM AMONG HEALTH PROFESSIONALS AND KNOWLEDGE REGARDING T&CM

The study also investigates the association between use/referral of T&CM and knowledge regarding T&CM: Knowledge was categorized into good knowledge and poor knowledge. The overall knowledge on T&CM among the health professionals was poor (61.2%). It is supported by other study that general practitioners' knowledge levels in CAM were low (60.8%) (Ozcakir et al. 2007).

With regards to the knowledge on T&CM, it was significantly higher in the HDOK (52.0%) than other hospitals (p=0.001). Multivariable analysis revealed that HDOK was 3.2 times, HPJ was 2.8 times, HSNZ was 1.7 and SGH was1.25 times more likely to have good knowledge regarding T&CM than UKMMC.

Non-Malay health professionals have higher knowledge (44.0%) than Malays (35.0%) regarding T&CM (p=0.047). Meanwhile, pharmacists have higher knowledge (47.2%) than nurses (37.9%) and doctors (32.5%) (p=0.03).

As far as the use of T&CM and knowledge regarding T&CM are concerned, although there were no significant relationship between use of T&CM and knowledge regarding T&CM, multivariable analysis revealed that health professionals who have good knowledge regarding T&CM were 1.6 times more likely to refer T&CM to their patients/family members in their whole life than health professionals who have poor knowledge regarding T&CM (p= 0.01).

Moreover, health professionals who have good knowledge regarding T&CM were 1.9 times more likely to refer acupuncture during their whole life (p=0.046).

Multivariable analysis showed that health professionals who have good knowledge regarding T&CM were 1.7 times and 1.9 times more likely to use herbal medicine in their whole life and in the last one year respectively than health professionals who have poor knowledge regarding T&CM (p=0.029 and p=0.038, respectively).

About half of them (51.0%) believed in the efficiency of CAM, whereas 38.0% did not. GPs desire more information about herbal medicine and acupuncture (Ozcakir et al. 2007).

Overall knowledge regarding T&CM among health professionals is low. Knowledge regarding T&CM was higher among the health professionals in HDOK than other four hospitals. It is very low among health professionals in UKMMC because UKMMC is not a T&CM integrated hospital. Non-Malay health professionals and pharmacists have higher knowledge on T&CM when compared to Malay health professionals and nurses and doctors respectively. There was no significant association between knowledge and use of T&CM. T&CM referral was higher among health professionals who have good knowledge regarding T&CM. Health professionals who have good knowledge regarding T&CM were more likely to refer acupuncture during their whole life and more likely to use herbal medicine.

ASSOCIATION BETWEEN USE OF T&CM AMONG HEALTH PROFESSIONALS AND ATTITUDE TOWARDS T&CM

The study also investigates the association between use/referral of T&CM and attitude towards T&CM; The attitude was categorized into positive attitude and negative attitude

PRACTICE OF TRADITIONAL AND
COMPLEMENTARY MEDICINE AMONG HEALTH
PROFESSIONALS IN MALAYSIA

towards T&CM. Majority of the respondents have positive attitude towards T&CM (65.4%).

In terms of attitude, positive attitude towards T&CM was high among health professionals in HSNZ (78.1%, p<0.001). Multivariable logistic regression indicates that HSNZ was three times (3.012 times), HDOK was almost three times (2.905 times) and HPJ and SGH were more than two times (2.251 and 2.127 times respectively) more likely to have positive attitude towards T&CM than UKMMC health professionals (p=0.003).

Statistical analysis revealed that health professionals aged 40 years old and above were 1.6 times more likely to have positive attitude towards T&CM than those below 40 years old (p=0.031).

Bivariate analysis showed that female health professionals have a more positive attitude towards T&CM (69.1%) than male health professionals (52.8%) (p=0.002).

Moreover, Malay health professionals showed higher positive attitude on T&CM (70.8%) than non-Malays (58.0%) (p=0.004). Multivariable analysis also supported that Malay health professionals were twice more likely to have positive attitude than non-Malay health professionals towards T&CM (p=0.007).

Muslim health professionals have higher positive attitude (70.5%) than non-Muslim health professionals (56.6%) towards T&CM (p=0.002).

In terms of career, nurses have higher positive attitude on T&CM (76.3%) than pharmacists (69.7%) and doctors (50.6%) (p<0.001). Multivariable analysis also showed that nurses were 3.1 times and pharmacists were 2.9 times more likely to have more positive attitude towards T&CM than doctors towards T&CM (p<0.001). This is in accordance with an early literature by Maida et al. (2008) who found that physicians have more negative attitude on T&CM compared to other health care professionals.

With regards to years of working, health professionals who have more than 10 years of working experience have higher positive attitude on T&CM (70.2%) than health professionals who have 10 years or less working experience (59.5%) (p=0.015). Health professionals who have diploma (74.8%) showed to have higher positive attitude than those with master or PhD (67.0%) and first degree (58.9%) (p=0.006).

Among the health professionals who have low income (RM<4000), 70.8% of them have positive attitude towards T&CM than the health professionals who have high income (RM≥4000) (59.4%), (p=0.009).

There is a relationship between use of T&CM and attitude towards T&CM. Health professionals who have positive attitude towards T&CM (51.9%) were more likely to use T&CM in their whole life than health professionals who have negative attitude towards T&CM (35.8%) (p=0.001). Statistical analysis were also revealed that health professionals who have positive attitude towards T&CM were 1.7 times and two times more likely to use T&CM during their whole life and in the last one year than health professionals who have negative attitude towards T&CM (p=0.006 and p=0.001, respectively). In contrast, a study reported that positive attitude towards CAM did not correlate with CAM referral (Maidi et al. 2008).

In term of relationship between referral of T&CM and attitude towards T&CM, health professionals who have positive attitude towards T&CM were two times more likely to refer T&CM than those who have negative attitude towards T&CM in their whole life (p<0.001) and almost three times (2.8 times) more likely to refer T&CM in the last one year (p<0.001).

Multivariable analysis revealed that health professionals who have positive attitude towards T&CM were more than two times (2.2 times) more likely to use massage (p=0.003) and almost 1.7 times more likely to refer massage than health professionals who have negative attitude towards T&CM during their whole life (p=0.022). The finding also revealed that health professionals who have positive attitude towards T&CM were 2.3 times more likely to refer massage than health professionals who have negative attitude towards T&CM in the last one year (p=0.005).

Health professionals who have positive attitude towards T&CM were two times more likely to refer acupuncture than health professionals who have negative attitude towards T&CM in their whole life and almost three times (2.87 times) more likely to refer acupuncture in the last one year (p=0.012).

Health professionals who have positive attitude towards T&CM were 1.7 times more likely to use herbal medicine compared to the health professionals who had negative attitude towards T&CM in their whole life. Health professionals who have positive attitude towards T&CM were almost three times (2.956) more likely to use herbal medicine than those who had negative attitude towards T&CM in the last one year (p=0.013).

Health professionals who had positive attitude towards T&CM were more than three times (3.2 times) more likely to refer patients/family to herbal medicine than those who had negative attitude towards T&CM in their whole life (p=0.006). Statistical analysis revealed that health professionals who have positive attitude towards T&CM were 6.7 times more likely to refer herbal medicine than health professionals who have negative attitude towards T&CM in the last one year (p=0.011).

There was no relationship between the use of postnatal care and attitude towards T&CM. Findings of this study revealed that health professionals who have positive attitude towards T&CM were 2.2 times more likely to refer postnatal care to their patients/family than health professionals who have negative attitude towards T&CM in their whole life (p=0.027).

However there was no relationship between the use of other types of T&CM and attitude towards T&CM. Statistical analysis revealed that health professionals who have positive attitude towards T&CM were 4.6 times more likely to refer other types of T&CM to their patients/family than health professionals who have negative attitude towards T&CM in their whole life (p=0.015) and more than three times (3.3

times) more likely to refer other types of T&CM than health professionals who have negative attitude towards T&CM in the last one year. Descriptive analysis indicates that 73.0% of health professionals believed that doctors should have knowledge about T&CM.

Positive attitude towards T&CM was high among the health professionals especially the health professionals in HSNZ and HDOK. Positive attitude towards T&CM was low in UKMMC as compared to other hospitals. This is probably because UKMMC is not a T&CM-integrated hospital. Positive attitude towards T&CM was high among senior staff, female, Malay, Muslim, nurses, health professionals who have 10 years or more working experience, health professionals who are holding diploma and health professionals with low income. Health professionals who have positive attitude towards T&CM were more likely to use T&CM and refer T&CM to their patients/family.

ASSOCIATION BETWEEN USE OF T&CM AMONG HEALTH PROFESSIONALS AND PERCEPTION ABOUT EDUCATION/ TRAINING IN T&CM

The study also investigates the association between use/referral of T&CM and perception about education/training in T&CM. The perception was categorized into positive perception and negative perception. A positive perception on education in T&CM was 85.3%.

Female health professionals have higher positive perception about education/training in T&CM (88.1%) than male health professionals (75.9%) (p=0.002).

In terms of career, pharmacists have higher positive perception (93.7%) about education/training in T&CM than nurses (86.4%) and doctors (77.1%) (p<0.001).

There was no significant association between use of T&CM and perception about education/training in T&CM.

Milden & Stokols (2004) and Winslow & Shapiro (2002) revealed that 60% and 80% physicians expressed interest in learning more about CAM in the US.

Ozcakir et al. (2007) reported that most of their physicians (96.5%) had not received any education about CAM but wanted to learn more (74.4%) and more than half of the GPs (62.7%) agreed with the necessity for CAM education.

A total of 21.4% have ever attended some T&CM classes or courses during their study, and 14.5% have joined workshops or conferences in T&CM, and 18.2% said education and training influenced their practice of T&CM.

About 89 % of the respondents agreed that educational materials about T&CM should be made available at their library and bookstores. It also showed that a total of 83.4% of the respondents agreed that T&CM practitioners have to learn conventional medicine, and that the perception about education in T&CM was highly positive among the health professionals.

PRACTICE OF TRADITIONAL AND COMPLEMENTARY MEDICINE AMONG HEALTH PROFESSIONALS IN MALAYSIA

REASON FOR PRECTICING AND NOT PRACTICING T&CM

Half of the T&CM users used T&CM to maintain their health and more than one third of health professionals used T&CM for both reasons (to maintain health and to treat health problems) while only 11.3% used because of health problem. Nearly half of the health professionals who recommended T&CM do so because of both reasons, one third of health professionals recommended T&CM to maintain health and only 17.2% health professionals recommended because of health problems.

Out of 211 (46.3%) health professionals who used T&CM, half of them (50.2%) said they used T&CM to maintain their health, and out of 232 (48.3%) health professionals who referred T&CM, less than half of them (38.3%) said they did so because of both reasons (to maintain health and to treat health problem). Meanwhile, more than half of the GPs (51.4%) believed in the efficiency of CAM (Ozcakir et al. 2007). In a study in England, White et al. (1997) reported that the majority of GPs believed that complementary medicine is effective.

Less than half of the health professionals (44.7%) used or recommended T&CM because they believed it was effective. One third of the health professionals (33.2%) said that they were satisfied with T&CM and 28.6% of the respondents believed it had fewer side effects.

Most of the health professionals (64.5%) have not used T&CM because they were not familiar with T&CM. Only 3.2% were dissatisfied with T&CM, while 3.9% of them stated that T&CM is a failure.

One third of the health professionals (34.6%) used or recommended T&CM to their patients and families because of their personal experience, followed by family's advice (30.4%), and by friend's or colleague's advice (26.2%).

FACTORS INFLUENCING THE T&CM USE/ RECOMMENDATION

Approximately one-third of the health professionals (34.6%) Used or recommended T&CM because of their own personal experience and one-third of them (30.4%) used or recommended T&CM because of family advice. A small number of health professionals (9.6%) used or recommended T&CM because of patients' opinion.

The most significant barrier for using or recommending T&CM to their patients and family among the health professionals were not being familiar with T&CM, potential side effects and drug-herb interaction.

Kurtz et al. (2003) supported that lack of evidence for effectiveness, potential side effects and interaction with allopathic treatments were the main barrier of not using CAM.

STRENGTH OF THE STUDY

The strength of the study lies in the combination of qualitative and quantitative studies. This study uses multiple approaches in data collection by using questionnaire in quantitative study and in-depth interviews in qualitative study. Another strength of the study is to be able to collect data from both east and west Malaysia.

STUDY LIMITATION

As this study uses self-administered questionnaire and in-depth interview, it is opened to information bias. The results obtained in this study should not be generalized to all the use of T&CM, since the study has only been carried out among the health professionals in five selected hospitals and among limited number of participants. Therefore, the results of this study might not reflect the use of T&CM among all the health professionals in Malaysia.

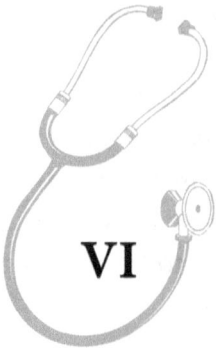

VI

CONCLUSION AND RECOMMENDATIONS

CONCLUSION

A cross-sectional study was carried out via quantitative and qualitative methods in five selected hospitals in West and East Malaysia. The study revealed that there was not a small numbers of health professionals used T&CM or referred T&CM to their patients and families. Knowledge regarding T&CM was poor in this study because most of the health professionals have never attended any T&CM classes/courses or workshops/conferences in their life. It turned out that most of the health professionals have positive attitude towards T&CM, but many have not been exposed to T&CM education, and most of the health professionals have positive perception about education/training in T&CM. They believed in the importance of education and training in T&CM for health professionals and agreed that it should be incorporated into medical faculty's curriculum.

PRACTICE OF TRADITIONAL AND COMPLEMENTARY MEDICINE AMONG HEALTH PROFESSIONALS IN MALAYSIA

The practice of massage, herbal medicine and postnatal care were higher than the use of acupuncture and other types of T&CM. Massage and acupuncture referral were higher than postnatal care, herbal medicine and other types of T&CM. Fewer health professionals used T&CM or recommended T&CM to their patients and families for health reasons while most of the T&CM users used it to maintain their health and most health professionals recommended T&CM because of both reasons.

The reason why one portion of the health professionals did not use or recommend T&CM was because they were not familiar with T&CM and afraid of T&CM side effects as well as drug-herbs interactions. Meanwhile, the reason why another portion of health professionals used or recommended T&CM was because they were satisfied with T&CM and due to its effectiveness.

Traditional and Complementary Medicine (T&CM) is becoming increasingly popular worldwide. It is the most invaluable treasure and has been developed over the course of thousands of years in the quest for human wellbeing. T&CM becomes a spotlight of society all over the world. A survey showed that a large percentage of the population (69.4%) used T&CM in their life and more than half of the population (55.6%) used T&CM in the last one year in Malaysia.

There is a growing interest in T&CM among the general population, and many patients increasingly seek information on T&CM therapies from health professionals. However, knowledge regarding T&CM among the health professionals is still lacking. Therefore, health professionals must have some basic knowledge about T&CM before they could offer advice to their patients. Doctors are of the utmost important in this regard because they play a very important role in patient care.

Though vast literature exists on the use of T&CM among the health professionals, the diversity of the questionnaire items made it challenging to summarize the findings. Despite this inclusive findings show that there is a growing interest and a desire by health professionals to obtain more information about T&CM.

Providing T&CM education to health professionals may help to integrate T&CM into the mainstream medicine. There are more than 11 universities in Malaysia that offer some form of medical education in T&CM and 14 government hospitals in Malaysia have T&CM units so far. However, knowledge regarding T&CM is still lacking not only among the health professionals in the not T&CM-integrated hospital, but also among the health professionals in T&M-integrated hospitals.

The use of T&CM among the general population and patients is widespread. Therefore, the attitude of health professionals towards T&CM is very important. Using health professionals also seems to be increasingly interested in T&CM.

Malaysia now therefore needs to have a traditional medical education system since T&CM has not been included in the curriculum of medical schools at the moment. Given the ultimate goal of healthcare is to improve patients' health, an increase in the health professionals' knowledge regarding

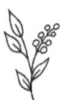

PRACTICE OF TRADITIONAL AND COMPLEMENTARY MEDICINE AMONG HEALTH PROFESSIONALS IN MALAYSIA

T&CM may help to rapidly integrate T&CM into the mainstream (western) medicine.

Knowledge regarding T&CM among health professionals is not as widespread as the public would demand it. Sound researches on T&CM effectiveness are needed to guide physicians' behavior, to protect patients' safety, and to assist policy-makers in planning regulations for T&CM usage. Most of the debate on T&CM focused on its safety and effectiveness. Unfortunately proper scientific evidences are lacking for most forms of T&CM.

Health professionals are aware of the importance of the subjects and wanted to learn more about T&CM and improve their knowledge. It would be reasonable to provide training opportunities for health professionals, primarily for the types of T&CM demanded by the population and recommended by the doctors. Many health professionals do not know whether they should use T&CM or not. Some of them tend to care about their patients using T&CM the same way as they would perceive the risk of consuming alcohol or cigarettes.

Although there have been several studies about T&CM conducted in other countries, unfortunately there are very limited studies regarding the use of T&CM and the reasons affecting the use of T&CM among the health professionals in Malaysia. This can be due to lack of knowledge and education and legal or cultural differences.

Malaysia is a tropical country and one of the richest countries in the world, with about 15,000-20,000 plant species based on the geographical evidence of the country (Taha et al. 2013).

Among them 1,300 species possessed medicinal values (Jamal 2006).

The use of different types of massage mainly Malay massage, herbal medicine and Malay postnatal care has become part of cultural tradition. Like other countries' traditional medicine, T&CM in Malaysia has been inherited from generation to generation and help to preserve the general health.

Herbal remedies are easily available from spice shops and herbalists without any regulatory control neither supervision in Malaysia. However, herbal medicine and other types of T&CM remedies have a lot of health benefits, but on the other hand, are not devoid of many harmful side-effects and possible drug-herb interactions. That is why, health professionals especially doctors must be aware of T&CM effectiveness and adverse effects, drug-herb interactions as well as toxicity of the T&CM remedies. Therefore, health professionals should have adequate knowledge regarding T&CM.

In this study, many health professionals requested for educational materials about T&CM to be made available at their library and bookstores and also they were willing to provide future training in T&CM for medical students. An integration of T&CM in undergraduate studies is beneficial for future health professionals to have some basic knowledge about T&CM. It is a very beneficial for the health professionals' personal improvement in knowledge regarding T&CM. At the same time, T&CM practitioners can be attached to health professionals to learn conventional medicine. It is good for T&CM practitioners to understand the mechanisms of disease clearly to improve and widen their knowledge. Because of the non-familiarity with T&CM, some health professionals are not in the position to practice or recommend T&CM.

Patients have the right to have access to T&CM as part of their cultural heritage and belief system. They should be given a choice in deciding whether to seek modern medicine or T&CM. health professionals' knowledge and attitude regarding T&CM are very important for guiding their patients. It is beneficial to integrate T&CM into Western Medicine and it would be useful for the Malaysian health care system.

RECOMMENDATIONS

1. **The study provides further evidence for sustaining the use of T&CM and T&CM referral among health professionals during their whole life and in the last one year. The findings imply the extent of present status of use of T&CM and T&CM referral and the associated factors influencing the current use of T&CM. The use of T&CM, T&CM referral and knowledge regarding T&CM are not as high as that found in some other studies, but the attitude towards T&CM is high. Yet, many health professionals wanted to learn about T&CM. Further studies are recommended to investigate trends regarding the practice of T&CM and its associated factors not only among health professionals but also among patients and the general population.**

2. We should understand the gap between the widespread acceptance of T&CM among the general public and its apparent neglect by the health professionals in order solve this problem.

3. Future research should be more focused on how to effectively integrate T&CM into the mainstream medicine effectively. We should have a clear picture on how the integration of T&CM could be successfully implemented in Malaysia.

4. Some components of T&CM should be part of a future curriculum for medical students. We should provide some opportunity for health professionals to have some basic knowledge about T&CM and make them feel comfortable in referring and counseling the patients with regards to T&CM service. By having this, we can provide and assure the patients with the comfort of safety treatments.

5. Ministry of Health (MOH) and the Ministry of Higher Education (MOHE) should encourage and support both public and private medical universities and colleges to include T&CM curriculum in fulfillment of their basic medical degree requirement.

6. It is time for the MOH to look into the current status of and policy on T&CM to determine and formulate the safe and effective way to integrate T&CM into other hospitals in Malaysia.

REFERENCES

Abdelwahab, S. I., Mohan, S., Elhassan, M.M., Al-Mekhlafi, N., Mariod, A.A., Abdul, A.B., Abdulla, M.A. & Alkharfy. K.M. 2011. Antiapoptotic and Antioxidant Properties of Orthosiphon stamineus Benth (Cat's Whiskers): Intervention in the Bcl-2-Mediated Apoptotic Pathway. *Evidence-Based Complementary and Alternative Medicine.* 2011:156765.

Abuduli, M., Ezat, Sh. & Aljunid, S. 2011. Role of traditional and complementary medicine in universal coverage. *Malaysian Journal of Public Health Medicine MJPHM.* 11 (2): 1-5.

Abuduli, M., Isa, Z. Md. & Aljunid, S.M. 2015. The gap between knowledge and perception on education in traditional and complementary medicine among medical staff in Malaysia. *Malaysian Journal of Public Health Medicine.* 15 (1): 77-82.

Abu-Irmaileh, B.E. & Afifi, F.U. 2003. Herbal medicine in Jordan with special emphasis on commonly used herbs. *J Ethnopharmacol.* 89(2-3):193–7.

Academy of Science Malaysia. 2011. A Mega-Science framework for sustained national development (2 0 1 1 – 2 0 5 0) Sustaining Malaysia's Future The Mega Science Agenda.

Affendy, H., Aminuddin, M., Azmy. M., Azimi, M. A., Assis, K. & Tamer, A. T. 2011. Effect of organic fertilizers application to the growth of orthosiphon stamineus benth entercropped with hevea brasiliensis willd. And Durio zibethinus Murr. *International Journal of Agricultural Reseacrh.* 6: 180-187.

Aggarwal, B.B., Kumar, A., Bharti, A.C. 2003. Anticancer potential of curcumin: preclinical and clinical studies. *Anticancer Res.* 23 (2003). 363–398.

Ahmed, T. & Gilani, A. H. 2009. Inhibitory effect of curcuminoids on acetylcholinesterase activity and attenuation of scopolamine-induced amnesia may explain medicinal use of turmeric in Alzheimer's disease. *Pharmacology Biochemistry Behavior* 91(4).

Ahmed, S., Anuntiyo, J., Malemud, C.J. & Haqqi, T.M. 2005. Biological Basis for the Use of Botanicals in Osteoarthritis and Rheumatoid Arthritis: A Review. *Evidence-Based Complementary and Alternative Medicine.* 2(3). 301-308.

Al Shaar, I.A.M.S., Ismail, M.F.S., Yousuf, W.A.A.A. & Salama, R.E. 2010. Knowledge, attitudes and practice of general practitioners towards complementary and alternative medicine in Doha, Qatar. *EMHJ.* 16 (5).

Ali, M.F., Abdul Aziz, A.F., Rashid, M.R.,Che Man, Z., Amir, A.A., Shien, L.Y., Ramli, N.Sh. & Abidin, N.A.A.Z. 2015. Usage of Traditional and Complementary Medicine (T&CM): Prevalence, Practice and Perception among Post Stroke Patients Attending Conventional Stroke Rehabilitation in A Teaching Hospital in Malaysia. *Med J Malaysia. 70 (1)*:18-23.

Amirghofran, Z. 2012. Herbal Medicines for Immunosuppression. *Iran J Allergy Asthma Immunol June.* 11(2): 111-119.

Ang, HH. & Sim, MK. 1997. Eurycoma longifolia Jack enhances libido in sexually experienced male rats. *Exp Anim.* 46(4): 287-90.

Arullappan, S., Rajamanickam, P., Thevar, N. & Kodimani, C.C. 2014. In *Vitro* Screening of Cytotoxic, Antimicrobial and Antioxidant Activities of Clinacanthus nutans (Acanthaceae) leaf extracts. *Tropical Journal of Pharmaceutical Research.* 13 (9): 1455-1461.

Aschwanden, C. 2001. Herbs for health, but how safe are they? *Bulletin of the World Health Organization* 79 (7): 691-692.

Aziz, R. A., Sarmidi, M. R., Kumaresan, S., Taher, Z. M. & Foo, D.C.Y. 2013. Phytochemical processing: the next emerging field in chemical engineering - aspects and opportunities. *Jurnal Kejuruteraan Kimia Malaysia.* 3. 45-60.

Aziz, Z. & Tey, N.P. 2009. Herbal medicines: Prevalence and predictors of use among Malaysian adults. Complementary therapies in medicine. *Complement Ther Med* 17 (1): 44-50.

Azizan, N.A., Ahmad, R., Mohamed, K., Ahmad, M.Z. & Asmawi, Z. 2012. The in vivo antihypertensive effects of standardized methanol extracts of Orthosiphon stamineus on spontaneous hypertensive rats: A preliminary study. *African Journal of Pharmacy and Pharmacology.* 6(6). 376 – 379.

Back Pain Facts and Statistics. 2008. American Chiropractic Association.

Barnes, P.M., Bloom, B. & Nahin, R.L. 2008. Complementary and alternative medicine use among adults and children. United States: National Center for Health Statistics.

Berman, BM., Singh, BB., Hartnoll, SM., Singh, BK. & Reilly, D.1998. Primary care physicians and complementary-alternative medicine: training, attitudes and practice patterns. *J Am Board Fam Pract.* 11: 272-281.

Biçen, C. Erdem, E. Kaya, C. Karatas, A., Elver, O. & Akpolat, T. 2012. Herbal Product Use in Patients with Chronic Kidney Disease. *Turkish Nephrology, Dialysis and Transplantation Journal.* 21(02): 136-140.

Bonakdar, R.A. 2002. Herbal Cancer Cures on the Web: Noncompliance With the Dietary Supplement Health and Education Act. *Fam Med.* 34(7): 522-7.

Borrelli, F., Capasso, R., Aviello, G., Pittler, MH. & Izzo AA. 2005. Effectiveness and safety of ginger in the treatment of pregnancy-induced nausea and vomiting. *Obstet Gynecol.* 105(4): 849-56. PMID: 15802416.

Bhowmik, D., Kumar, K.P.S. Tripathi, P. & Chiranjib.B. 2009. Traditional Herbal Medicines: An Overview. *Archives of Applied Science Research.* 1 (2) 165-177.

Bouldin, A. S., Smith, M.C., Garner, D.D, Szeinbach, Sh.L., Frate, A.A. & Croom. E.M. 1999. Pharmacy and herbal medicine in the US. *Social Science & Medicine.* 49 (1999) 279±289.

Boucher, T.A. & Lenz, S.K. 1998. An organizational survey of physicians: attitudes about and practice of complementary and alternative medicine. *Altern Ther.* 4: 59-64.

Buettner, C., Kroenke, C.H., Phillips, R.S., Davis, R.B. & Eisenberg, D.M. 2006. Correlates of use of different types of complementary and alternative medicine by breast cancer survivors in the nurses' health study. *Breast Cancer Res Treat* 100: 219–227.

Buono, M.D., Urciuoli, O., Marietta, P., Padoani, W. & Leo, D.D. 2001. Alternative medicine in a sample of 655 community-dwelling elderly. *J Psychosom Res.* 50: 147–154.

Burke, A., Upchurch, D.M., Dye, C. & Chyu, L. 2006. Acupuncture use in the United States: findings from the

National Health Interview Survey. *J Altern Complement Med.* 12: 639–648.

Catherine, E. & Ulbricht. 2010. Natural Standard Herb & Supplement Guide: An Evidence-Based Reference. Mosby *Elsevier.* 527. Missouri, USA. 2010. Hardback. ISBN: 978-0-323-07295-3.

Cem, B. Sahin, A.S & Sahin, T.K. 2013. A survey of Turkish hospital patients' use of herbal medicine. *European Journal of Integrative Medicine.* 5 (2013) 547–552.

Chang, L.C., Huang, N., Chou, Y.J., Lee, C.H. & Kao, F.Y. 2008. Utilization patterns of Chinese medicine and Western medicine under the National Health Insurance Program in Taiwan, a population-based study from 1997 to 2003. *BMC Health Serv Res.* 8: 170.

Chattopadhyay, I., Biswas, K., Bandyopadhyay, U., Banerjee, R.K. 2004. Turmeric and curcumin: Biological actions and medicinal applications. *Current Science.* 87:(1) 44-50

Chaudhury, R.R. & Rafei, U.M. 2001. Traditional medicine in Asia. World health organization regional office for South-East Asia, New Delhi: SEARO Regional Publications. No. 39.

Chagan, L., Bernstein, D., Cheng, J., Kirschenbaum, H., Rozenfeld, V., Caliendo, G., Meyer, J. & Mehl, B. 2005. Use of biological based therapy in patients with cardiovascular diseases in a university-hospital in New York City. *BMC Complementary and Alternative Medicine* 5 (1): 4.

Chen, F.P., Chen, T.J., Kung, Y.Y., Chen, Y.C. & Chou, L.F. 2007. Use frequency of traditional Chinese medicine in Taiwan. *BMC Health Serv Res.* 7: 11.

Chen, J.X. & Hu, LS. 2006. Traditional Chinese medicine for the treatment of chronic prostatitis in China: a systematic review and meta-analysis. *J Altern Complement Med.* 12: 763-769.

Ching, S.M., Zakaria, Z.A., Paimin, F. & Jalalian, M. 2013. Complementary alternative medicine use among patients with type 2 diabetes mellitus in the primary care setting: a cross-sectional study in Malaysia. *BMC Complementary and Alternative Medicine.* 13:148. DOI: 10.1186/1472-6882-13-148.

Choi, H. K., Kim, D. H., Kim, J.W., Ngadiran, S., Sarmidi, M.R. & Park, C.S. 2010. Labisia pumila extract protects skin cells from photoaging caused by UVB irradiation. *Journal of Bioscience and Bioengineering.* 109 (3) 291-296.

Choi, Y.D., Xin, Z.C. & Choi, H.K. 1998. Effect of Korean red ginseng on the rabbit corpus cavernosal smooth muscle. *International Journal of Impotence Research.* 10 (1) p37. 7p.

Chui, P.L., Abdullah, K. L., Wong, L.P. & Taib, N. A. 2014. Prayer-for-health and complementary alternative medicine use among Malaysian breast cancer patients during chemotherapy. *BMC Complement Altern Med.* 14: 425.

Chung, V., Wong, E., Woo, J., Lo, S.V. & Griffiths, S. 2007. Use of traditional Chinese medicine in the Hong Kong special administrative region of China. *J Altern Complement Med.* 13: 361–367.

Cohen, I., Tagliaferri, M. & Tripathy, D. 2002. Traditional Chinese Medicine in the Treatment of Breast Cancer. Seminars in Oncology. *Science Direct.* 29 (6) 563–574.

Corbin, W.L. & Shapiro, H. 2002. Physicians want education about complementary and alternative medicine to enhance communication with their patients. *Arch Intern Med.* 162 (10): 1176-1181.

Clement, Y.N., Williams, A.F., Khan, K., Bernard, T., Bhola, S., Fortun, M., Medupe, O., Nagee, K. & Seaforth, C.E. 2005. A gap between acceptance and knowledge of herbal remedies by physicians: the need for educational intervention. *BMC Complementary and Alternative Medicine.* 5 (1): 20.

Cruez, A.F. 2007. Traditional medicine in Malaysia. http://forums.hpathy.com/forum.

Daly, M., Tai, Ch.J., Deng, Ch.Y. & Chien, L.Y. 2009. Factors associated with utilization of traditional Chinese medicine by white collar foreign workers living in Taiwan. *BMC Health Services Research.* 9: 10.

Dahlui, M. & N.A. Aziz. 2012. 'Developing health service hub in ASEAN and asia region country report on healthcare service industry in Malaysia'. in Tullao,

T.S.and H.H.Lim(eds.), Developing ASEAN Economic Community (AEC) into A Global Services Hub, ERIA Research Project Report 2011-1, Jakarta: ERIA. 65-110.

Damião, C.M., Francisco, J.D.S., Débora, R.L.S., Cláudia, L.V. & Ana M.C.G. 2002. Seroepidemiological markers of enterically transmitted viral hepatitis A and E in individuals living in a community located in the North Area of Rio de Janeiro, RJ, Brazil. *Mem Inst Oswaldo Cruz, Rio de Janeiro.* 97(5): 637-6.

Dans, AM., Villarruz, MV., Jimeno. CA., Javelosa, MA., Chua. J., Bautista. R. & Velez. GG. 2007. The Effect of Momordica Charantia Capsule Preparation on Glycemic Control in Type 2 Diabetes Mellitus Needs Further Studies. *Journal of Clinical Epidemiology.* 60(6): 554-9.

Davis, M.P. & Darden, P.M. 2003. Use of complementary and alternative medicine by children in the United States. *Arch Pediatr Adolesc Med.* 157: 393–396.

Dhanoa, A., Yong, T. L., Yeap, S.J.L., Lee, I.H. Z. & Singh, V. A. 2014. Complementary and alternative medicine use amongst Malaysian orthopaedic oncology patients. *BMC Complement Altern Med.* 14: 404.

Duke, J.A. 2002. Hand book of medicinal herbs. (2nd ed.) CRC Press. ISBN 9780849312847 - CAT# 1284.

Duvoix, A., Blasius, R., Delhalle, S., Schnekenburger, M., Morceau, F. & Henry, E et al. 2005. Chemopreventive and therapeutic effects of curcumin. *Cancer Lett,* 223 181–190

Eisenberg, D.M., Davis Davis, R.B., Ettner S.L, Appel, S., Wilkey, S., Van Rompay, M. & Kessler, R.C. 1998. Trends in alternative medicine use in the United States, 1990-1997: results of a follow-up national survey. *JAMA.* 280: 1569-75.

Ernst, E. & Resch, K-L. 1995. White AR: Complementary medicine. What physicians think of it: a meta-analysis. Arch Intern Med. 155: 2405-8.

Eurycoma longifolia. Wikipedia, the free encyclopedia.

Fadzil, F., Anuar, HM., Ismail, S., Ghani A.N. & Ahmad, N. 2012. Urut Melayu, the traditional Malay massage, as a complementary rehabilitative care in postpartum stroke. *J Altern Complement Med.* 18(4): 415-9.

Fountain-Polley, S., Kawai, G., Goldstein, A. & Ninan, T. 2007. Knowledge and exposure to complementary and alternativemedicine in paediatric doctors: a questionnaire survey. *BMC Complementary and Alternative Medicine.* 7 (1): 38.

Fuangchan, A., Sonthisombat, P., Seubnukarn, T,. Chanouan, R., Chotchaisuwat, P., Sirigulsatien, V., Ingkaninan, K., Plianbangchang, P. & Haines, ST. 2011. Hypoglycemic Effect of Bitter Melon Compared With Metformin in Newly Diagnosed Type 2 Diabetes Patients. *Journal of Ethnopharmacology.* 134(2): 422-8.

Fujiwara, K., Imanishi, J., Watanabe, S., Ozasa, K. & Sakurada, K. 2011. Changes in attitudes of Japanese doctors toward complementary and alternative medicine-comparison of surveys in 1999 and 2005 in Kyoto. *Evidence-based Complementary and Alternative Medicine.* ID 608921,7.

Ghasemzadeh, A., Nasiri, A., Jaafar, H.Z., Baghdadi, A. & Ahmad, I. 2014. Changes in Phytochemical Synthesis, Chalcone Synthase Activity and Pharmaceutical Qualities of Sabah Snake Grass (*Clinacanthus nutans* L.) in Relation to Plant Age. *Molecules.* 19(11):17632-17648.

Ghazali, F.CH. 2009. IFM surface profiler, μCT 3D SCAN, and electron microscopical investigation of 'Sanggul Fatimah' (Anastatica Hierochuntica L) MC. Volume 2. *Life science.*

Giannelli, M., Cuttini, M., Da Frè, M. & Buiatti, E. 2007. General practitioners' knowledge and practice of complementary/alternative medicine and its relationship with life-styles: a population-based survey in Italy. *BMC Fam Pract.* 15; 8:30.

Gray, R.E., Fitch, M., Goel, V., Franssen, E. & Labrecquem, M. 2003. Utizilation of complementary/alternative services by women with breast cancer. *J Health Soc Policy.* 16:75–84].

Gonzalez, A.E. Stuart. Prickly Pear Cactus ('Nopal') for the Treatment of Type 2 Diabetes Mellitus. Chapter 46. Bioactive Food in Chronic Diseases States. Bioactive Food as Dietary Intervention for Diabetes. 601.

Gordon, N.P., Sobel, D.S. & Tarazona, E.Z. 1998. Use of and interest in alternative therapies among adult primary care clinicians and adult members in a large health maintenance organization. *West J Med.* 169: 153-161.

Gunjan, M., Naing, T.W., Saini, R.S. Ahmad, Ab. Naidu, J.R & Kumar, I. 2015. Marketing trends & future prospects of herbal medicine in the treatment of various disease. *World Journal of Pharmaceutical Research.* 4(9) 132-155.

Harmsworth, K. & Lewith, G.T. 2001. Attitudes to traditional Chinese medicine amongst western trained doctors in the People's Republic of China. *Social science & medicine* 52 (1): 149-53.

Hanssen, B., Grimsgaard, S., Launsø, L., Fønnebø, V. & Falkenberg, T. 2005. Use of complementary and alternative medicine in the Scandinavian countries. *Scand J Prim Health Care* 23: 57–62.

Herman, C.J., Dente, J.M., Allen, P. & Hunt, W.C. 2006. Peer reviewed: Ethnic differences in the use of complementary and alternative therapies among adults with osteoarthritis. *Preventing Chronic Disease.* 3 (3): 1-15.

Hishikawa, N., Takahashi, Y., Amakusa, Y., Tanno, Y., Tuji, Y., Niwa, H., Nobuyuki, M. & Krishna. UK. 2012. Effects of turmeric on Alzheimer's disease with behavioral and psychological symptoms of dementia. *Ayu.* 33 (4): 499–504.

Huang, N., Chou, Y.J., Chen, L.S., Lee, C.H., Wang, P.J. & Tsay, J.H. 2011. Utilization of western medicine and traditional Chinese medicine services by physicians and their relatives: The role of training background. *Evidence-based Complementary and Alternative Medicine.* 827979,7 10.1093.

Ibrahim, M. H., Jaafar, H.Z.E., Rahmat, A. & Rahman, Z.A. 2011. Effects of Nitrogen Fertilization on Synthesis of Primary and Secondary Metabolites in Three Varieties of Kacip Fatimah (*Labisia Pumila* Blume). *Int. J. Mol. Sci.* 12(8), 5238-5254.

"Kacip Fatimah (Labisia Pumila)". Jefferson Griuen. 2008. Wikipedia. Free encyclopedia.

Kamat, A.M., Sethi, G., Aggarwal, B.B. 2007. Curcumin potentiates the apoptotic effects of chemotherapeutic agents and cytokines through down-regulation of nuclear factor-kappa B and nuclear factor-kappaB-regulated gene products in IFN-alpha-sensitive and IFN-alpha-resistant human bladder cancer cells. *Mol Cancer Ther.* 6 (2007). 1022–1030.

Khatun, M. A., Harun-Or-Rashid, Md. & Rahmutulla, M. 2011. Scientific Validation of Eight Medicinal Plants Used in Traditional Medicinal Systems of Malaysia: a Review. *American-Eurasian Journal of Sustainable Agriculture.* 5(1): 67-75.

Kim, M., Han, H.R., Kim, K.B. & Duong, D.N. 2002. The use of traditional and Western medicine among Korean American elderly. *J Community Health.* 27: 109–120.

Koumpouros, Y. & Birbas, K. 2013. Use of information and communication technologies (icts) to support diffusion of traditional medicine across european and asian countries: the greek perspective. *Health Science Journal.* 7 (4).

Kuttan, R., P. Bhanumathy., K. Nirmala., M.C. George. 1985. Potential anticancer activity of turmeric (Curcuma longa). *Cancer Letters.* 29: (2) 197-202. Elsevier.

Jamal, J.A. 2006. Malay traditional medicine: An overview of scientific and technological progress. Special Feature: Traditional medicine: *S&T Advancement. Tech Monitor.*

Jamal, J.A. et al. 2004. "Perkembangan Penyelidikan and Perkembangan Kacip Fatimah (translation: Advancements in Research and Development of Kacip Fatimah)". New Dimensions in Complementary Health. Forest Research Institute of Malaysia: 13–19.

Jantan, I. 2004. Medicinal Plant Research in Malaysia: Scientific Interests and Advances IBRAHIM. *Jurnal Sains Kesihatan Malaysia* 2(2) 27-46.

Johnson, T., Boon, H., Jurgens, T., Austin, Z., Moineddin, R., Eccott, L. & Heschuk, S. 2008. Canadian pharmacy students' knowledge of herbal medicine. *American journal of pharmaceutical education.* 72 (4).

Harmsworth, K.G.T. Lewith. 2001. Attitudes to traditional Chinese medicine amongst western trained doctors in the People's Republic of China. *Social Science and Medicine.* 52: 149-153.

Holtz, C. 2007. Global health care: Issues and policies. Sudbury, MA: Jones & Bartlett Publishers.

Hwa, JB., Suk, KH. & Jong, CS. 2000. Effect of Saponin and Non-saponin of Panax Ginseng on the Blood Pressure in the Renovascular Hypertensive Rats. *Journal of Ginseng Research*. Labisia Pumila. Wikipedia. The free encyclopedia. 23 (2): 99 81-87.

Ikram R.R.R. and Ghani, M.K.A. 2015. An Overview of Traditional Malay Medicine in the Malaysian Healthcare System. *Journal of Applied Sciences*. 15: 723-727.

Lai, D. & Chappell, N. 2007. Use of traditional Chinese medicine by older Chinese immigrants in Canada. *Fam Pract*. 24: 56–64.

Lazareto, D.M.M. 2011. Study protocol exercise background document, European programme for intervention epidemiology training.

Lee, C. H. & Kim, J.H. 2014. A review on the medicinal potentials of ginseng and ginsenosides on cardiovascular diseases. *Journal of Ginseng Research*. 38(3) 161–166.

Lee, P.Y., Taha, A.B.A., LIN, K., Ghazali, S.R., Syed Ahmad, S.H. & Almashoor. 2007. Usage of complementary and alternative medicine among primary attendees, Kuching, Sarawah, Malaysia. *Asia Pecific Journal of Family Medicine*. 6 (1).

Lee, S.H., Cekanova, M. & Baek, S.J. 2007. Multiple mechanisms are involved in 6-gingerol-induced cell growth arrest and apoptosis in human colorectal cancer cells. *Molecular Carcinogenesis.* 47(3): 197-208.

Lee, S.I., Khang, Y.H., Lee, M.S. & Kang, W. 2002. Knowledge of, attitudes toward, and experience of complementary and alternative medicine in western medicine and oriental medicine-trained physicians in Korea. *American journal of public health.* 92 (12): 1994-2000.

Levine, S.M., Weber-Levine, M. & Mayberry, R.M. 2003. Complementary and Alternative Medical Practices: Training, Experience and Attitudes of a Primary Care Medical School Faculty. *J Am Board Fam Pract.* 16: 318-26.

Leung, L., Birtwhistle, R., Kotecha, J., Hannah, S., & Cuthbertson, S. 2009. Anti-diabetic and hypoglycaemic effects of *Momordica charantia* (bitter melon): a mini review. British Journal of Nutrition. 102 (12). 1703-1708.

Liao, G-S., Apaya, M K. & Shyur, L-F. 2013. Herbal Medicine and Acupuncture for Breast Cancer Palliative Care and Adjuvant Therapy. *Evid Based Complement Alternat Med.* 2013 (2013). 437948.

Liu F, Li ZM, Jiang YJ, Chen LD. 2014. A Meta-Analysis of Acupuncture Use in the Treatment of Cognitive Impairment After Stroke. *J Altern Complement Med.* 20(7): 535–544.

Leung, L., Birtwhistle. R., Kotecha. J., Hannah. S., & Cuthbertson, S. 2009. Anti-Diabetic and Hypoglycaemic Effects of Momordica Charantia (Bitter Melon): A Mini Review. *British Journal of Nutrition*.

Lewith GT, Hyland M, Gray SF. 2001. Attitudes to and use of complementary medicine among physicians in the United Kingdom Complementary Therapies in Medicine. Complement. *Ther Med.* 9(3): 167-72.

Loh, C.H. 2009. Use of traditional Chinese medicine in Singapore children: perceptions of parents and paediatricians. *Singapore Med J.* 50: 1162–1168.

Lim, J., Wong, M., Chan, M.Y., Tan, A.M., Rajalingam, V., Lim, L.P., Lou, J. & Tan, C.L. 2006. Use of complementary and alternative medicine in paediatric oncology patients in Singapore. *Annals-Academy of Medicine Singapore.* 35 (11): 753.

Malay pantang: hot compress. Baby Center. www.babycenter.com.my › For You › Asian confinement › Traditional confinement.

Malaysia. Confederation of Asia Pacific Chambers of Commence and Industry.

Malaysia. 2016. Wikipedia, the free encyclopedia.

Manneräs, L., Fazliana, M., Wan Nazaimoon, W.M., Lönn, M., Gu, H.F., Ostenson, C.G. & Stener-Victorin, E. 2009. Beneficial metabolic effects of the Malaysian herb

Labisia pumila var. alata in a rat model of polycystic ovary syndrome. *Journal of Ethnopharmacology.* 127 (2). 346–351.

MacPherson, H., Sinclair-Lian, N. & Thomas, K. 2006. Patients seeking care from acupuncture practitioners in the UK: a national survey. *Complement Ther Med.* 14: 20–30.

Milden, S.P. & Stokols, D. 2004. Physician's attitudes and practices regarding complementary and alternative medicine. *Behavioral Medicine.* 30: 73-82.

Mills, E., Jacques, J., Perri, D.D. & Koren, G. 2006. Herbal medicines in pregnancy and lactation an evident based approach. Taylor & Francis Medical, an imprint of the Taylor & Francis Group 0-41537-392-1.

Ministry of Health Malaysia. 2009. Traditional and Complementary Medicine Practice Guidelines on Herbal Therapy as Adjunct Treatment for Cancer. First Edition. Traditional and Complementary Medicine Division Ministry of Health Malaysia.

Mishra, S. & Palanivelu. K. 2008. The effect of curcumin (turmeric) on Alzheimer's disease: An overview. *Annals of Indian Academy of Neology.* 11(1). 13-19.

Mohamed, E.A.H., Mohamed A.J., Asmawi, M.Z., Sadikun, A., Ebrika, O.S. & Yam M.F. 2011. Antihyperglycemic Effect of Orthosiphon Stamineus Benth Leaves Extract and Its Bioassay-Guided Fractions. *Molecules.* 16(5), 3787-3801.

Mohd Zin, M.H. 2009. Traditional and complementary medicine in Malaysia. T&CM report. Malaysian Medical Association. ISSN: 0216-71-40 PP1285/12/2009 (023006) MITA (P) 123/1/91.

Molassiotis, A.l., Fernadez-Ortega, P., Pud, D., Ozden, G., Scott, J.A., Panteli, V., Margulies, A., Browall, M., Magri, M., Selvekerova, S., Madsen, E., Milovics, L., Bruyns, I., Gudmundsdottir, G., Hummerston, S., Ahmad, A.M., Platin, N., Kearney, N & Patiraki, E. 2005. Use of complementary and alternative medicine in cancer patients: A European survey. *Ann Oncol.* 16:655-63.

Molly, M.R. & Xiaorui, Z. 2011. The world medicines situation 2011 traditional medicines: Global situation, issues and challenges. Geneva: *World Health Organization.*

Morris, KT., Johnson, N., Homer, L., & Walts, D. 2009. A comparison of complementary therapy use between breast cancer patients and with other primary tumor sites. *Am J Surg.* 179:407–11.

Mullaichairam, A.R. 2011. Counterfeit herbal medicine. *International Journal of Nutrition, Pharmacology, Neurological Diseases.* 1 (2): 97-102.

Nabeel, G. M. & Hassan. G. A. 2005. Ginger Lowers Blood Pressure Through Blockade of Voltage-Dependent

Calcium Channels. *Journal of Cardiovascular Pharmacology.* 45(1) 74-80.

Nadkarni, K. M. 2007. Indian materia medica with Ayurvedic, Unani-Tibbi, Siddha, Allopathic, Homeopathic, Naturopathic & Home Remedies, Appendices & Indexes. Volume 2. Popular Prakashan.

National Policy of Traditional and Complementary Medicine. 2001. http:// tcm.moh.gov.my/v4/ pdf/ National Policy. Pdf.

Oberbaum, M., Notzer, N., Abramowitz, R. & Branski, D. 2003. Attitude of medical students to the introduction of complementary medicine into the medical curriculum in Israel. *The Israel Medical Association Journal: IMAJ.* 5 (2): 139-42.

Odugbemi, T. 2008. A textbook of medical plants from Nigeria. ISBN: 978-978-48712-9-7: 1-61.

Oguamanam, C. 2008. Patents and traditional medicine: Digital capture, creative legal interventions, and the dialectics of knowledge transformation. *Indiana Journal of Global Legal Studies.* 15 (2): 489-528.

Okojie. L.O. & Orisajimi. O.S., 2011. Valuation of the recreational benefits of Old Oyo National Park, Nigeria: A travel cost method analysis. *Journal of Food, Agriculture & Environment.* 9 (1): 521-525.

Omonona, B.T., Egbetokun, O. A., Ajijola, S. & Salaam, A. H. 2012. Consumer preference for medicinal plants in Oyo

Metropolis, Nigeria. *Journal of Medicinal Plants Research.* 6(20):3609.

Ong, H.C, Ruzalila, B.N & Milow, P. 2011.Traditional knowledge of medicinal plants among the Malay villagers in Kampung Tanjung Sabtu, Terengganu, Malaysia. *Indian Journal of Traditional Knowledge.* 10 (3). 460-465.

Ozcakir, A., Sadikoglu, G., Bayram, N., Mazicioglu, M.M., Bilgel, N. & Beyhan, I. 2007. Turkish general practitioners and complementary/alternative medicine. *The Journal Of Alternative And Complementary Medicine* 13 (9): 1007–1010.

Pan, C., Huo, Y., An, X., Singh, G., Chen, M., Yang, Z., Pu J. & Li J. 2012. Panax notoginseng and its components decreased hypertension via stimulation of endothelial-dependent vessel dilatation. *Vascular Pharmacology.* 56 (3–4). 150–158.

Pandey, M.M., Rastogi, S. & Rawat, A.K. 2008. Indian herbal drug for general healthcare: An overview. *The Internet Journal of Alternative Medicine.* 6 (1) ISSN: 1540-2584.

Pal, S.K. & Shukla, Y. 2003. Herbal medicine: current status and the future. *Asian Pacific J Cancer Prev.* 4: 281-288.

Peninsular Malaysia 2016. Wikipedia, the free encyclopedia.

Payyappalliman, U. 2009. Role of traditional medicine in primary health care: An overview of perspectives and challenges. *Yokohama Journal of Social Sciences.* 14 (6): 58-75.

Planta, M., Gundersen, B. & Petitt, J.C. 2000. Prevalence of the use of HP in a low-income population. *Family Medicine.* 32: 252–257

Pu, C.Y., Lan, V.M., Lan, C.F. & Lang, H.C. 2008. The determinants of traditional Chinese medicine and acupuncture utilization for cancer patients with simultaneous conventional treatment. *Eur J Cancer Care.* 17: 340–349.

Ragozin, B. V. 2016. The history of the development of Ayurvedic medicine in Russia. Anc Sci Life. 35(3): 143–149.

Ramsewak, R.S., DeWitt, D.L. & Nair, M.G. 2000. Cytotoxicity, antioxidant and anti-inflammatory activities of Curcumins I–III from Curcuma longa. *Phytomedicine.* 7 (4). 303-308.

Reed, P. & Wu, Y. 2013. Logistic regression for risk factor modelling in stuttering research. *J Fluency Disord.* 38(2): 88-101.

Rees, R.W., Feigel, I., Vickers, A., Zollman, C., Mc Gurk, R. & Smith, C. 2000. Prevalence of complementary therapy use by women with breast cancer: a population based survey. *Eur J Cancer.* 36:1354–64.

Reynaldo, J. & Santos, A. 2009. Cronbach's Alpha: A Tool for Assessing the Reliability of Scales. Vol. 37 (2). Tools of the Trade. 2TOT3.

Rhode, J., Fogoros, S., Zick S., Wahl, H., Griffith, K.A., Huang, J. & Liu J.R. 2007. Ginger inhibits cell growth and modulates angiogenic factors in ovarian cancer cells. *BMC Complementary and Alternative Medicine.* 7:44.

Roberson. E. 2008. Medicinal Plants at Risk. Nature's Pharmacy, Our Treasure Chest: Why We Must Conserve Our Natural Heritage. *A Native Plant Conservation Campaign Report.*

Riccard, C.P. & Skelton, M. 2008. Comparative analysis of 1st, 2nd, and 4th year MD students' attitudestoward complementary alternative medicine (CAM). *BMC Research Notes.* 1: 84.

Sabry, W.M & Vohra, A. 2013. Role of Islam in the management of Psychiatric disorders. *Indian J Psychiatry.* 55(Suppl 2): S205–S214.

Safarzadeh, E., Shotorbani, S.S. & Baradaran, B. 2014. Herbal Medicine as Inducers of Apoptosis in Cancer Treatment. *Adv Pharm Bull.* 4 (Suppl 1): 421–427.

Saleh, J. & Machado, L. 2012. Rose of Jericho: A Word of Caution. *Oman Med J.* 27(4): 338. doi: 10.5001/omj.2012.86. PMCID: PMC3464751.

Samuels, N., Zisk-Rony, R.Y., Singer, S.R., Dulitzky, M., Mankuta, D., Shuval, J.T. & Oberbaum, M. 2010. Use of and attitudes toward complementary and alternative medicine among nurse-midwives in Israel. *American Journal of Obstetrics and Gynecology.* 203 (4): 341.e1-341.e7.

Sawni, A. & Thomas, R. 2007. Pediatricians' attitudes, experience and referral patterns regarding complementary/alternative medicine: a national survey. *BMC Complementary and Alternative Medicine.* 7 (1): 18.

Sekar, M. & Rashid, N.A. 2016. Formulation, Evaluation and Antibacterial Properties of Herbal Ointment Containing Methanolic Extract of Clinacanthus nutans Leaves. *International Journal of Pharmaceutical and Clinical Research.* 8 (8): 1170-1174

Sewitch, M.J., Cepoiu, M., Rigillo, N. & Sproule D. 2008. A literature review of health care professional attitudes towards complementary and alternative medicine. *Complementary Health Practice Review.* 13: 139.

Shapiro, K. & Gong, W.C. 2002. Natural Products Used for Diabetes. *Journal of the American Pharmaceutical Association.* 42 (2) 217-226.

Shrivastava, S. Dube. D., Kapoor, Dubey, P. 2007. "The Pharmacist's Role in Herbal Care" *Medscape.*

Shuid, A. N., Ping, L. L., Muhammad, N., Mohamed, N. 2011. The Effects of Labisia pumila var. alata on bone markers and bone calcium in a rat model of post-menopausal osteoporosis. Journal of Ethnopharmacology. 133 (2011) 538–542.

Stavro, PM., Woo M. & Vuksan, V. 2004. P-2: Korean red ginseng lowers blood pressure in individuals with hypertension. *American Jnl of Hypertension.* 17 (S1). Pp. 33A.

Subramaniam, D. S. S. 2013. Health minister: 12pc deaths in government hospitals due to cancer. www.themalaymailonline.com/.../health-minister-12pc-deat.

Suekawa, M., Ishige, A., Yuasa, K., Sudo, K., Aburada, M. & Hosoya. E. 1984. Pharmacological Studies On Ginger. I. Pharmacological Actions Of Pungent Constituents, (6)-Gingerol And (6)-Shogaol. *Journal of Pharmacoblo-Dynamics.* 7 (11) P836-848.

Shuid, A.N., Ping, L.L., Muhammad, N. Mohamed, N., Soelaiman, I.N. 2011. The effects of Labisia pumila var. alata on bone markers and bone calcium in a rat model of post-menopausal osteoporosis. *Journal of Ethnopharmacology.* 33:(2) 538–542. http://dx.doi.org/10.1016/j.jep.2010.10.033.

Shih, C.C., Su, Y.C., Liao, C.C. & Lin, J.G. 2010. Patterns of medical pluralism among adults: results from the 2001 National Health Interview Survey in Taiwan. *BMC Health Serv Res.* 10: 191.

Shih, S.F., Lew-Ting, C.Y., Chang, H.Y. & Kuo, K.N. 2008. Insurance covered and non-covered complementary and alternative medicine utilization among adults in Taiwan. *Soc Sci Med.* 67: 1183–1189.

Shih, Y.T., Hung, Y.T., Chang, H.Y., Liu, J.P. Lin, H.S. 2003. The design, contents, operation and the characteristics of the respondents of the 2001 National Health Interview Survey in Taiwan. *Taiwan J Public Health.* 22: 419–430.

Shmueli, A. & Shuval, J. 2004. Use of complementary and alternative medicine in Israel: 2000 vs. 1993. *Isr Med Assoc J.* 6: 3–8.

Sooi, L.K. & Keng, S.L. 2013. Herbal Medicines: Malaysian Women's Knowledge and Practice. *Evidence-Based Complementary and Alternative Medicine.* 438139, 10 doi: 10.1155/2013/438139.

Srivastava, KC. & Mustafa, T. Ginger (Zingiber officinale) and rheumatic disorders. *Med Hypothesis.* 29 (1989): 25-28.

Srivastava, KC. & Mustafa, T. 1992. Ginger (Zingiber officinale) in rheumatism and musculoskeletal disorders. *Med Hypothesis.* 39(1992): 342-8.

Sikand, A. & Laken, M. 1998. Pediatricians' experience with and attitudes toward complementary/alternative medicine. *Arch Pediatr Adolesc Med.* 152: 1059–1064.

Siti, Z.M., Tahir, A., Farah, AI., Fazlin, SMA., Sondi, S., Azman, AH & Zaleha, WCW. 2009. Use of traditional and complementary medicine in Malaysia: a baseline study. *Complement Ther Med.* 17(5–6): 292–299.

Stange, R., Amhof, R. & Moebus, S. 2008. Complementary and alternative medicine: attitudes and patterns of use by German physicians in a national survey. *TheJournal of Alternative and Complementary Medicine*. 14 (10): 1255-1261.

Suhami, N., Muhamad, M. & Krauss, S.E. 2014. The Islamic Healing Approach to Cancer Treatment in Malaysia. *Journal of Biology, Agriculture and Healthcare*. 4(6). 104-110.

Sustainable Consumption. 2008. Academic conference proceedings. Edina Vadovics & Emese Gulyás (eds.). Sustainable consumption. Budapest, Hungary.

Taha, H., Arya, A. Mohd, M.A. & Hadi, A.H.A. 2013. Bioactive Compounds of Some Malaysian Annonaceae Species. 4th International Conference on Advances in Biotechnology and Pharmaceutical Sciences (ICABPS' 2013) 12-13. Singapore.

Taid, T. C. & Rajkhowa, R. C. & Kalita, J.C. 2014. A study on the medicinal plants used by the local traditional healers of Dhemaji district, Assam, India for curing reproductive health related disorders. *Advances in Applied Science Research*. 5(1):296-301

Talbott, S.M., Talbott, J.A., George, A. & Pugh, M. 2013. Effect of Tongkat Ali on stress hormones and psychological mood state in moderately stressed subjects. *J Int Soc Sports Nutr*. 10: 28.

Tam, A., Chan, M.L.D. & Suki, N.M. 2014. Understanding consumption of the traditional and complementary medicine: a conceptual model. *International Journal of Research in Management & Social Science*. 2 (3) (V). 1-6.

Tavakoli, J., Miar, S., Zadehzare, M.M & Akbari, H. 2012. Evaluation of Effectiveness of Herbal Medication in Cancer Care: A Review Study. Iran J Cancer Prev. 5(3): 144-156.

The role of service in the tourism and industry. www.thestar.com.my.

The telegraph. Malaysia bans Muslims from practicing yoga. 2008.

Thomas, K., Nicholl, J. & Coleman, P. 2001. Use and expenditure on complementary medicine in England: a population based survey. *Complement Ther Med*. 9: 2–11.

Traditional Chinese Medicine Could Make "Health for One" True. www.who.int/intellectualproperty/studies/Jia.pdf.

Tilburt, J.C. & Kaptchuk, T.J. 2008. Herbal medicine research and global health: an ethical analysis. *Bulletin of the World Health Organization*. 86: 594-599.

Tindle, H., Davis, R., Phillips, R. & Eisenberg, D. 2005. Trends in use of complementary and alternative medicine by US adults: 1997-2002. *Altern Ther Health Med*. 11: 42-49.

Traditional and Complementary Medicine Division. 2011. A handbook of Traditional and Complementary Medicine in Malaysia. tcm.moh.gov.my/v4/pdf/handbook.pdf

UNESCO. 2010. Draft preliminary report on traditional medicine and its ethical implications. United Nations Educational, Scientific and Cultural Organization Internal Bioethic Committee (IBC).

Upchurch, D.M., Burke, A., Dye, C., Chyu, L. & Kusunoki, Y. 2008. A socio behavioral model of acupuncture use, patterns, and satisfaction among women in the United States, 2002. *Women Health Issues.* 18: 62–71.

VanderCreek, L., Rogers, E. & Lester, J. 1998. Use of alternative therapies among breast cancer outpatients compared with the general population. *Altern ther health med.* 5:71–6.

Verma, Sh. & Singh, SP. 2008. Current and Future status of Herbal medicines. *Veterinary World.* 1 (11): 347-350.

Vinjamury, S. P., Vinjamury, M., Claudia der Martirosian and Judith Miller. 2014. Ayurvedic Therapy (*Shirodhara*) for Insomnia: A Case Series. *Glob Adv Health Med.* 3(1): 75–80.

What is Misai Kucing? "Let thy food be thy medicine…" Hippocrates the Father of Medicine.

WHO. 2002. Traditional medicine strategy 2002-2005. Geneva: *World Health Organization.*

WHO. 2000. General guidelines for methodologies on research and evaluation of traditional medicine. Geneva: World Health Organization.

WHO. 2001. Traditional medicine strategy 2002-2005. Geneva: World Health Organization.

WHO. 2000. Development of national policy on traditional medicine. Geneva: World Health Organization Western Pacific Region.

WHO. 2010. Report. Informal meeting on strategic direction on traditional medicine in the western pacific region. World health organization regional office for western pacific region. Manila, Philippines.

WHO. 2005. WHO global atlas of traditional, complementary and alternative medicine. World Health Organization. Vol. 1.

Wigler, I., Grotto, I., Caspi, D. & Yaron, M. 2003. The effects of Zintona EC (a ginger extract) on symptomatic gonarthritis. Osteoarthritis Cartilage. 11(11): 783-9.

Winslow, C.L. & Shapiro, H. 2002 Physicians want education about complementary and alternative medicine to enhance communication with their patients. Achieves of Internal Medicine. 162: 1176-1181.

Wright. S.H. 2012. Perceptions of factors related to therapeutic change in face to face and distance counseling environments. Counseling and human services - Dissertations. Paper 54.

Wu, A.P., Burke, A. LeBaron, S. 2007. Use of traditional medicine by immigrant Chinese patients. *Fam Med.* 39: 195–200.

Xu, S. & Levine, M. 2008. Medical residents' and students' attitudes towards herbal medicines: a pilot study. *The Canadian journal of clinical pharmacology.* 15 (1).

Yatim, R. M., Muhamad, M., Krauss, S. E. & Lateef, A. 2015. Islamic Healing Use Among Malay-Muslim Cancer Patients: Malaysian Perspective. *Australian Journal of Asian Country Studies.*

Yeh, C.H., Tsai, J.L., Li, W., Chen, H.M., Lee, S.C., Lin. C.F. & Yang, C.P. 2000. Use of alternative therapy among pediatric oncology patients in Taiwan. *Pediatr Hematol Oncol.* 17: 55-65.

Yong YK., Tan JJ., Teh SS., Mah SH., Ee GC., Chiong HS. & Ahmad Z. 2013. Clinacanthus nutans Extracts Are Antioxidant with Antiproliferative Effect on Cultured Human Cancer Cell Lines. *Evid Based Complement Alternat Med.* 462751.

Zhang Z.J., Tan, Q.R., Tong, Y., Wang, X.Y. & Wang, H.H. 2011. An epidemiological study of concomitant use of Chinese medicine and antipsychotics in schizophrenic patients: implication for herb-drug interaction. *PLoS One.* 6: e17239.

www.ingramcontent.com/pod-product-compliance
Lightning Source LLC
Chambersburg PA
CBHW020741180526
45163CB00001B/306